Neonatal Lung Ultrasonography

Jing Liu • Erich Sorantin • Hai-Ying Cao
Editors

Neonatal Lung Ultrasonography

PMPH PEOPLE'S MEDICAL PUBLISHING HOUSE Springer

Editors
Jing Liu
Department of Neonatology and NICU
Beijing Chaoyang District Maternal and
Child Healthcare Hospital
Beijing, China

Erich Sorantin
Division of Pediatric Radiology
Department of Radiology
Medical University of Graz
Graz, Austria

Hai-Ying Cao
Department of Ultrasound
GE Healthcare
Beijing, China

Jointly published with People's Medical Publishing House, Beijing, China
ISBN 978-94-024-1547-6 ISBN 978-94-024-1549-0 (eBook)
https://doi.org/10.1007/978-94-024-1549-0

Library of Congress Control Number: 2018956410

This Springer imprint is published by the registered company Springer Nature B.V.
The registered company address is: Van Godewijckstraat 30, 3311 GX Dordrecht, The Netherlands

Preface

Neonates and premature babies represent the most vulnerable patient group owing to their limited ability to negotiate their "unfamiliar" life after delivery. Therefore, a special environment using incubators is set up to provide homeostasis, for example, temperature. "Minimal handling" is one of the major strategies in neonatology, and every action must be balanced between possible harms and benefits.

Almost 40 years have passed since the introduction of ultrasound in clinical use. Starting with obstetrics, many areas of the body can be scanned safely by ultrasound; the most common investigations involve abdominal, urinary tract, gynecological, and obstetric sonography as well as echocardiography. Children differ in many respects from adults, including in their psychology, communication, circulation, body composition, and proportions, to name just a few. Depending on age, a variable, usually considerable, amount of the skeleton is not calcified but consists of cartilage. This presents new challenges and possibilities for ultrasound. Owing to the reduced craniocaudal chest length compared to adults, the upper abdominal organs are less covered by the rib cage, and in combination with, for example, the small amount of intestinal fat content, high-quality images with excellent resolution can be obtained easily. In addition, Doppler ultrasound makes it possible to detect, monitor, and quantify flow. Therefore, challenging applications, like brain ultrasound and spinal or hip sonography, are possible. Even better, all investigations can be conducted bedside, including those involving the use of incubators, making ultrasound the perfect imaging tool in neonatology.

Considering the high frequency of lung diseases in premature babies due to their inherent immaturity, it is a logical step to evaluate and describe the potential of lung ultrasound. For several years chest ultrasound was used for the evaluation of pleural effusions, consolidation, surfactant deficiency states, and pneumothorax detection. Enthusiastic pediatricians and radiologists used ultrasound also to guide interventions and insertions of peripheral lines; in particular, correct, central positioning can be monitored noninvasively by ultrasound using a subcostal approach.

In children, Prof. Dr. Erich Sorantin has been applying ultrasound to all body regions for more than 30 years, and the challenges of lung ultrasound have always attracted him. Dr. Jing Liu and Hai-ying Cao were the first neonatologist and radiologist, respectively, to develop this technology in China under the auspices of Prof. Sorantin starting in 2011.They gained extensive experience in this field through long-term clinical practice with a large number of patients, so the time has come to promote this technology by means of a neonatal lung ultrasound monograph.

This book tries to close the gap between clinical needs and sporadic lung ultrasound publications. For the first time this book provides a comprehensive overview of several typical, neonatal lung diseases and includes pathophysiology and clinical findings in combination with lung ultrasound. Moreover, care was taken to embed lung ultrasound findings in the clinical management of vulnerable patients.

The book is intended to be read by physicians of all (sub)specialties interested in the imaging and management of neonatal lung diseases including neonatologists and pediatricians, pediatric radiologists, and intensive care and emergency room doctors. Furthermore, the authors believe strongly that using lung ultrasound will reduce the number of chest films in susceptible patients, thereby preventing their exposure to radiation and protecting them from the harmful effects of radiation.

We want to thank Dr. Clark Zhe Wu, professor at the University of Electronic Science and Technology of China, who provided much help in English editing and ultrasound physics. His invaluable assistance helped to improve the quality of the book.

Beijing, China — Jing Liu
Graz, Austria — Erich Sorantin
Beijing, China — Hai-Ying Cao
September 28, 2017

Contents

About the Editors

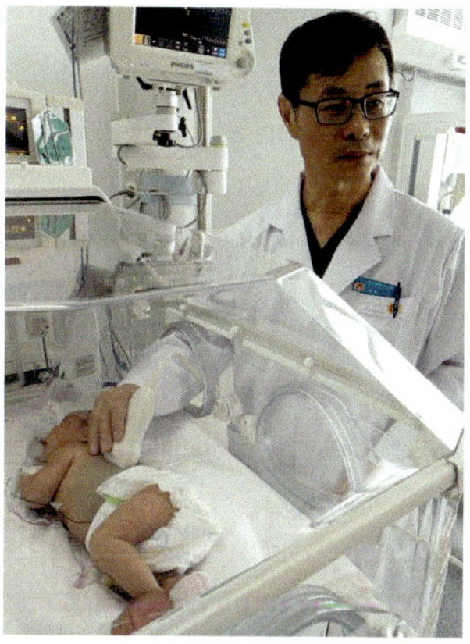

Jing Liu, Ph.D., M.D., is the Director of the Department of Neonatology and NICU, Beijing Chaoyang District Maternal and Child Health Care Hospital. He is skilled at neonatal intensive critical care and neonatal brain and lung ultrasound. His academic positions include Associate Chairman of Chinese Neonatologist Association, Chairman of the Specialized Committee on Chinese Maternal Origin Neonatal Disease Research, Associate Chairman of Beijing Neonatology Association, and Associate Chairman of Perinatal Medicine Section, Chinese Academy of Pediatrics. In addition, he is an editorial member of more than 20 Chinese and English journals. Dr. Jing Liu has published more than 280 papers, over 12 books, and book chapters. His research work has been supported by the China Natural Science Foundation, among other organization, and he has won 12 awards for science and technology granted by the government of China.

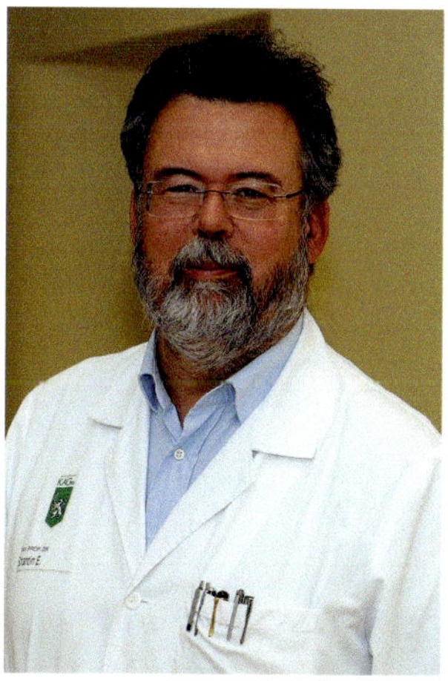

Erich Sorantin was born in 1957 and studied medicine at the Alma Mater Rudolfina in Vienna, Austria. After graduation he was trained as a general practitioner, followed by a full residency in pediatrics, and after switching to the Department of Radiology, Medical University Graz, he added another residency in radiology with a special focus on pediatric radiology. He obtained a professorship in 2002. Since 2013 he has served as acting head of the Division of Pediatric Radiology, Department of Radiology, Medical University Graz, Graz, Austria.

His scientific interests include, besides pediatric radiology, biocomputing, biosimulation, radiation protection, noninvasive imaging, signal and image processing, and artificial intelligence.

As a pediatrician he published a paper on computing neonatal mechanical ventilation. In 1995–1996 he led the first EC research project at the University of Graz in breast cancer detection and artificial intelligence. He served as consultant to Siemens for computer graphics for more than 10 years, and the virtual endoscopy part of two workstations was partly developed by him. Additionally, he introduced digital imaging for children at his institution. Moreover, he optimized Computed Tomography at the Medical University of Graz and several software applications for pediatric use. He also obtained a license as an ultrasound instructor.

He published and authored more than 300 papers, which have received 1244 citations and received 20 awards.

Furthermore, Dr. Sorantin is the network coordinator for a large-scale, multi-institutional, international network (www.ceepus.org) covering more than 40 academic institutions and organizing six summer/winter schools every year, in addition to supporting interdisciplinary research.

Dr. Sorantin has been married for more than 30 years and has three adult sons.

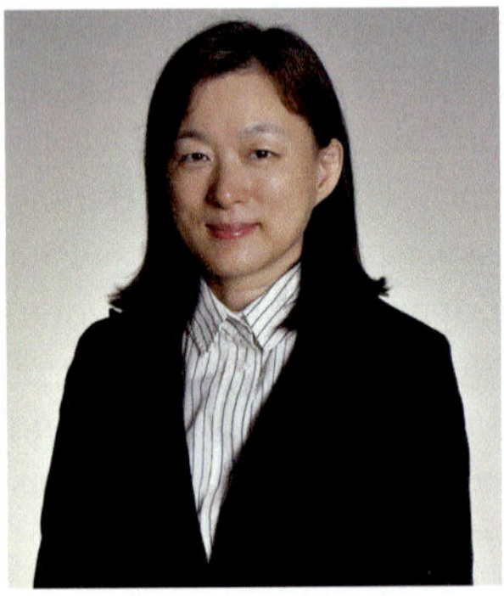

Hai-Ying Cao, M.D., has 10 years of experience as an ultrasound doctor and for more than 5 years served as direct of ultrasound department. Later, she joined GE Ltd. (China) specializing in clinical education or application. Dr. Hai-Ying Cao has extensive clinical experience and comprehensive skills and has coauthored several books and published almost 20 papers.

Introduction

Ultrasound is one of the most commonly used tools in clinical imaging. However, its potential application in diagnosing lung diseases has been restricted because the lung has always been considered an organ that is not amenable to ultrasound examination, generally because of the total reflection of ultrasound waves in encountering air. So far, chest X-rays or CT scanning is the first choice among the common diagnosing tools in lung diseases. But an extension of ultrasound practice to diagnosing, examining, and monitoring lung disease provides a novel and easier way through the "forbidden zone."

In detecting lung problems, lung ultrasound has proved to be more favorable in many aspects, including accuracy, reliability, convenience, simplicity, and safety, while its feasibility and convenience as a bedside application in neonatal intensive care unit add further appeal. The aim of this book is to introduce ultrasound imaging features with respect to newborn common lung diseases, such as respiratory distress syndrome, transient tachypnea of newborns, infectious pneumonia of newborns, meconium aspiration syndrome, pulmonary atelectasis of newborns, pulmonary hemorrhage, pneumothorax, and other clinical practices. The typical ultrasound images of the aforementioned lung diseases were organized in such a way as to provide a solid base of understanding and facilitate the use of the information presented. Furthermore, the fundamental principles, terminology, and scanning skills relevant to lung ultrasound will also be demonstrated in this book. It is the authors' belief that this book will achieve the goal of improving the application of lung ultrasound in this field.

1 The Basic Principles of Lung Ultrasound

Hai-Ying Cao and Erich Sorantin

With the progress and development of medical science, ultrasound has become an indispensable part of clinical work, and its applications are expanding. Originally considered to be unfeasible by many doctors [1, 2], lung ultrasound has been applied and is changing the neonatal intensive care treatment process. Real-time ultrasound can be used to evaluate the anatomy and dynamics of organs and hemodynamic information. This chapter introduces the basic principle and operation skills of two-dimensional and Doppler ultrasonography. It is convenient for doctors who have just started to use ultrasound to understand and master the use of sound instruments, scan and optimize images, and understand image information correctly.

Electronic Supplementary Material The online version of this chapter (https://doi.org/10.1007/978-94-024-1549-0_1) contains supplementary material, which is available to authorized users.

H.-Y. Cao (✉)
Department of Ultrasound, GE Healthcare, Beijing, China
e-mail: hai_ying.cao@china.med.ge.com

E. Sorantin
Division of Pediatric Radiology, Department of Radiology, Medical University Graz, Graz, Austria

1.1 Basic Principles of Ultrasound

1.1.1 Common Physical Quantities of Sound Waves

An ultrasonic wave refers to a wave with a frequency of over 20,000 Hz, beyond the human hearing range. Ultrasound is a mechanical wave, usually generated by a piezoelectric crystal in the transducer. The transducer acts as both the transmitter and the receiver. When the human body is scanned, the transducer-emitting sound waves are spread in the tissues, and then, the transducer receives the echo in the tissues. The detection and display of the reflected and scattered sound energy from the body constitute the basis of the diagnostic ultrasound. When the sound waves propagate in a completely uniform medium, the medium presents the echoless or cyst sign. The tissue contact surfaces of two different physical characteristics form an interface. This interface will reflect a certain amount of sound wave energy. The amount of reflected sound wave energy depends on the difference in acoustic impedance between the two tissues that form the interface. Acoustic impedance Z is defined as tissue density ρ multiplied by the acoustic wave propagation velocity in the tissue C, i.e., $Z = \rho C$. The difference in acoustic impedance between the two tissues that form the interface determines the strength of the echo signal; the greater the

J. Liu et al. (eds.), *Neonatal Lung Ultrasonography*, https://doi.org/10.1007/978-94-024-1549-0_1

impedance difference, the more energy is reflected back. For instance, in the tissue-air (chest-lung) interface, the difference in acoustic impedance is great, resulting in 99% of the sound waves being reflected back and no energy entering the tissue for further imaging. Therefore, when healthy lungs are scanned, the pulmonary sonogram shows homogeneous chaotic gray pictures; this is not a solid structure, and all signs arise from the pleural line [3]. For this reason as well, when the ultrasound scan is performed, the coupling gel is sprayed on the skin between the transducer and the scanning area so that there is no gas between the patient's skin and the transducer, and the acoustic wave energy can successfully enter the human tissues.

Ultrasound equipment performs the depth positioning of reflectors according to the return time of the wave sound. To generate two-dimensional images, the emission of a series of ultrasound pulses into the body tissues is needed. When the strength of the received echo signals is strong, it is manifested as bright on the monitor; when there is no signal, it is manifested as black. Therefore, the ultrasound images use different strengths or brightnesses to manifest the oscillator intensity of reflection signals.

1.1.2 Interaction Between Acoustic Sound and Tissues

The sound waves will experience a series of interactions such as attenuation, acoustic energy absorption, reflection, scattering, refraction, and diffraction during the propagation along the direction of scan lines when meeting the organs and tissues:

1. Attenuation: The acoustic wave will be absorbed, scattered, and reflected by tissues when disseminated in tissues, and energy will become attenuated. The attenuation degree depends on the frequency of the sound wave and the dielectric properties of sound waves. The higher the wave sound frequency is, the more attenuation there is; therefore, the frequency of the transducer determines the depth of the transducer and the amount of information that is obtained. The attenuation coefficient is not the same in different tissues. The attenuation coefficients of bones and air are approximately 5 and 12 dB/cm/MHz and that in the soft tissues is approximately 0.70 dB/cm/MHz. A black information-free area is often observed at the rear of skeletons, which we call acoustic shadow. When the neonatal lungs are scanned, acoustic shadow is behind the ribs and scapula. Attenuation has important clinical significance and can influence the selection of the transducer, time gain compensation, acoustic output, and system gain adjustment.
2. Acoustic energy absorption: During the acoustic wave propagation process in the tissue, part of its energy is absorbed by tissues, which is a major factor in sound energy attenuation. Thus, in the far field of the images, gain compensation is often used to ensure image consistency.
3. Reflection: Two kinds of media with different acoustic impedances cause some acoustic energy to return to the transducer and form an echo. Echo generation and detection are the foundation of ultrasound imaging. The mode of the ultrasound reflection on the interface between two media depends on the size and surface characteristics of the interface. When faced with a large and smooth interface, the reflected energy is very much as a mirror surface reflects light. At this time, we call it the specular reflection interface. In lung ultrasound examination, the diaphragm and pleura often become a specular reflection interface; when the insonation is perpendicular to the interface, the sound wave directly returns to the transducer, resulting in a brighter echo. Therefore, we should try to keep the insonation perpendicular to the structure of interest.

1.1.3 Color Ultrasound

Neonatal lung ultrasound examination can help identify whether or not the echo-free structure is a blood vessel and can simultaneously confirm whether it is an artery or vein as well as the blood flow direction. Color Doppler ultrasound has been widely used in clinical practice and becomes an indispensable meaningful technology in ultrasound clinical diagnosis. Color Doppler ultrasound characterizes the blood flow information within the selected regions with colors, and they are superimposed on the grayscale or tint images that represent the body's anatomical structure. Clinically, the blood flow information in the tissue region can often tell us whether the tissues in this region work normally. In neonatal lung examination, it will help us observe the blood flow characteristics of lungs after consolidation and obtain the hemodynamic parameters, such as velocity of flow and resistance indexes. Of course, the application of color Doppler is far greater than that.

The physical basis of color Doppler technology is the Doppler effect, i.e., when the scattering source is moved toward the transducer, the echo frequency becomes higher. If the scattering source is moved dorsally to the transducer, the backward wave frequency will become lower. The change in frequency is proportional to the moving speed of the scattering source. That is, if the frequency changes and some related parameters are known, we can back-deduce the movement speeds of the scattering source. This is the most fundamental physical basis of color Doppler imaging. Ultrasound machines encode the blood flow velocity and direction information with colors to obtain color images. Red and blue are usually used to express the blood direction toward and away from the probe. Under the color ultrasound, the relatively high pulse repetition frequency (velocity scale) and wall filter are adopted to avoid the color noise caused by faster respiration movements in fetuses.

1.1.4 Ultrasound Artifact

Ultrasound generates many artifacts because of its physical characteristics. Traditionally, when we study ultrasound diagnosis technology, it is important to learn how to recognize and avoid artifacts. Ultrasound image quality is probably more dependent than any other image mode on the skill of the operators to identify and avoid artifacts and traps. Artifacts are incorrect images, and the displayed structures on the images do not actually exist. Generally, artifacts are induced by the physical phenomenon that influences the sound beam propagation. Additionally, some artifacts are induced by defects in scan technology and the improper use of ultrasound devices. The former is unavoidable, but the latter is avoidable. To understand the artifacts, we will seriously consider some basic assumptions of ultrasound image formation [4]:

1. Transmitted waves travel in straight lines from the transducer.
2. The reflection on the structure is returned along the central axis of the sound beam.
3. The sound beam in the elevational direction is very, very thin.
4. The scattering intensity corresponds to the reflection intensity of the reflector, or the size of the amplitude of the sound wave is proportional to the size of the acoustic impedance among the tissues.
5. The propagation velocity of sound beams in tissues is the same, and the speed is accurate and constant, approximately 1540 m/s. The distance between the reflector and transducer footprint is proportional to the round-trip time of sound beams.
6. The acoustic wave directly reaches the reflectors and returns, and the path is the shortest.
7. The detected echo originates from the last ultrasound pulse.

In reality, they are not as assumed. These assumptions are not always true, and there are various exceptions. Acoustic wave characteristics, errors in scan technology, the wrong use of the device, or special anatomic structures can produce artifacts. During fetal lung scanning, we usually encounter reverberation, which is the cause of A-line and comet tail.

1. Reverberation: Reverberation artifacts originate from the special reflective interface and lead to repeated reflection to form the equidistant linear echoes. Contrary to other artifacts, we need to take full advantage of these artifacts for the diagnosis and differential diagnosis of lung diseases. When there are

highly reflective interfaces close to the site near the transducer surface, the incident sound waves meet the strong reflection interface, and the reflected echo returns to the transducer surface and again returns to human tissues. This sound wave reflects back and forth until the energy becomes attenuated. Ultrasound signal reflection occurs repeatedly, and there is a delayed signal that returns to the transducer. As shown in Figs. 1.1 and 1.2, the first pulse leaves the transducer and then meets the strong reflection interface. It reflects back to the transducer to form a short linear echo (E1); the remaining energy (sound wave 2) returns to the tissues, and a reflection similar to pulse 1 occurs and likewise forms a high echo (E2 then returns to the tissues to form echo E3). In the same way, in normal lungs, there are multiple high-amplitude reflections that come back and forth between the transducer and the strong reflection interface when the incident beam is perpendicular to the pleura. Additionally, there are linear echoes that are parallel with gradually decreasing intensity and equal spacing. When the beam is not perpendicular to the pleura, multiple reflections basically disappear (Fig. 1.3), so in the lung ultrasound scan, attempts should be made to make the sound beam perpendicular to the pleura to confirm the diagnosis of normal and abnormal lungs.

Because the pleura on the left side of the image is not perpendicular to the beam near the probe mark, no multiple reflections formed. On the opposite side of the image (right side of the image), we found parallel multiple line-like echoes from the near field to the far field because the beam in this area is perpendicular to the pleura.

2. Shadow: Shadow is defined as the reduction in the amplitude of echoes, which appears as a strip-shape anechoic zone (black) because most of the energy is reflected and absorbed. When we scan the neonatal lung longitudinally, the ribs will result in a shadow. When the compound technology is applied, the shadow will be weakened because the sound beam is from multiple directions, avoiding the bone or other highly reflective or absorbed structures. When the water in the lung increases enough to have a compact B line, the shadow will disappear.
3. Comet tails: A comet tail is a kind of reverberation artifact that appears as a trail of dense continuous echoes [5]. The comet-tail sign is produced only in small and strong reflection

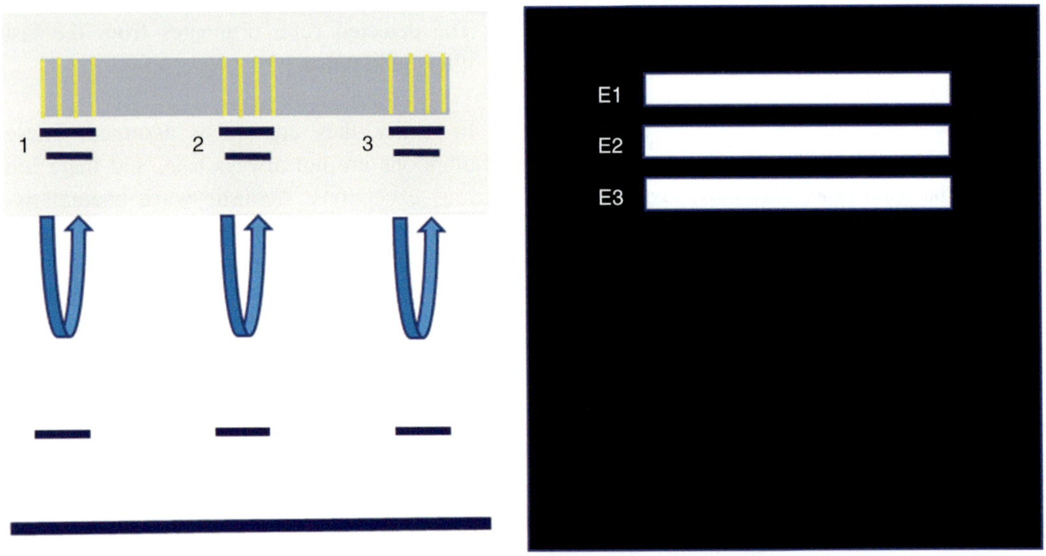

Fig. 1.1 Schematic diagram of the formation of reverberation artifacts

interfaces. Because there are two strong reflection interfaces, the ultrasound wave reflects back and forth between the two interfaces. Since the interfaces are very close, the formed echoes are also very close, and they are not distinguished from each other. The time delay of continuous multiple time points is interpreted as a distance. In addition, the surface of the hyperechoic reflector is not parallel to the probe surface, and much more reverberation pulses are reflected off in other directions, so the attenuation intensity gradually decreases, the width becomes gradually narrow, and their shape is triangular pyramidal. The shapes of the comet-tail sign are complex and various, depending on the target shape, component, size, scan direction, and distance from the transducer. The comet-tail sign is commonly found in an anechoic area, and such artifacts are common in lung ultrasound images of normal infants within 3 days after birth (Fig. 1.4).

4. Ring down and B-line: The ring-down effect was once considered to be a variant of the

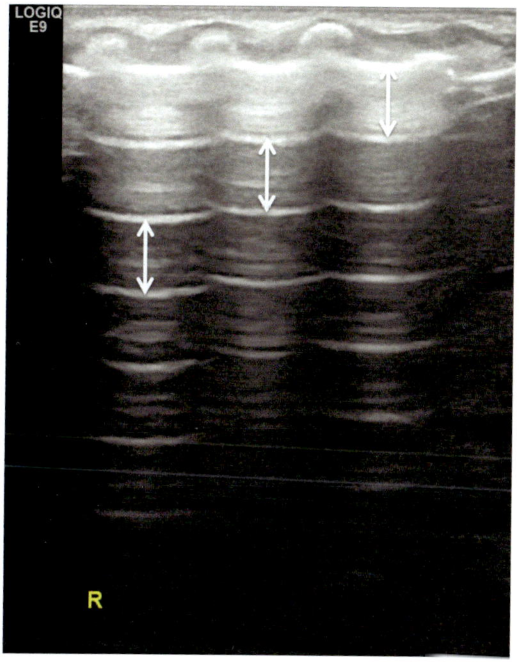

Fig. 1.2 As the depth increases, the intensity of the pleural line gradually decreases. The distances between the A-lines are equidistant and are equal to those between the transducer and the pleural line

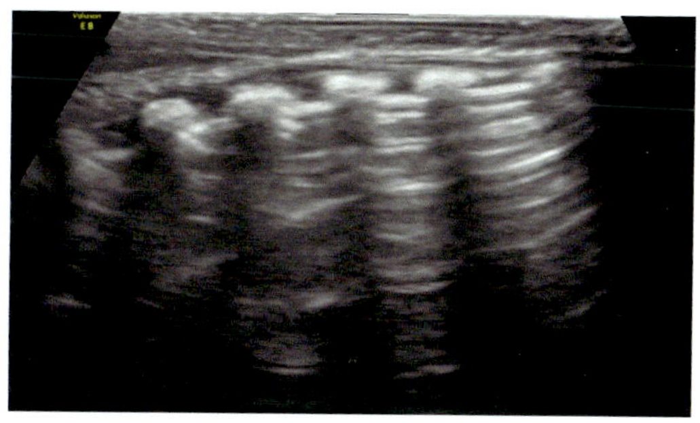

Fig. 1.3 Production of reverberation artifacts

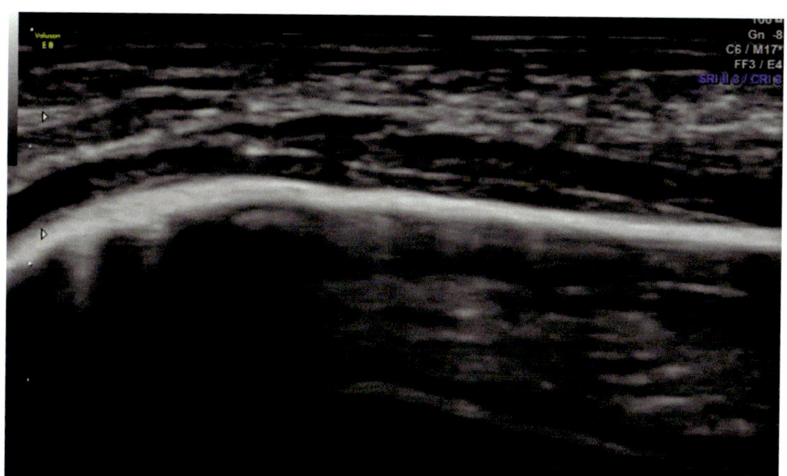

Fig. 1.4 Comet-tail sign (Video 1.1)

comet-tail sign because the two artifacts look similar but their causes are different. One single bubble and one layer of bubbles cannot produce a ring-down effect, but when there are two layers of bubbles, horn- or bugle-shaped fluid collection will form, and ring down will occur [6]. When pulmonary interstitial lesions occur, the ultrasound wave energy will cause the resonance of small amounts of liquid, which are trapped among four microbubbles. The continuous sound wave generated by this vibration will return to the transducer to excite the vibration crystals, generating a series of linear or a series of parallel linear echoes extending from the posterior direction of the gas to the depth without fading [6–8]. The ring down in the lungs is from the subpleural and intralobular interstitia or interlobular septa and fissure [9]. The B-line is a term to describe the ring-down effect and starts from the pleura in the lung ultrasound image.

1.2 The Optimization of the 2D Mode

For general ultrasound equipment, there is no specific preset for neonatal lung examination. Thus, one can select a small part preset or create new preset for neonatal lung scanning. When we scan the patient, we can optimize the image according to the needs and the patient's condition to obtain a satisfactory image.

1. Frequency: The operator usually can change the frequency according to the patient's situation to obtain a good image. On the basis of ensuring the penetration, try to select higher frequency to get the best quality. The higher the frequency of the transducer, the shorter the wavelength and spatial pulse length, which results in better image quality and more attenuation. When you decrease the frequency, the penetration will improve. To maintain the balance of the resolution and penetration, the ultrasound frequency of the probe for neonatal lung diagnosis is between 9 and 14 MHz.
2. Focus numbers and position: When the frequency is changed, the axial resolution is mainly affected. To improve the lateral resolution, we can use focus to decrease the beam width to improve lateral resolution. Move the focus to the area of interest. To obtain a good resolution image, you can use multiple focuses, but more focuses will decrease the frame rate.
3. Dynamic range and compression: The ratio of the strongest amplitude and the lowest amplitude is called the dynamic range, which can be displayed on the screen and expressed in decibels (dB). In typical clinical applications, the range of reflected signals ranges from 1 to 1012, so the maximum dynamic range is 120 dB. Although the amplifier of the ultrasonic instrument can handle these signals, the maximum signal intensity that the grayscale can express is only 35–40 dB, so the dynamic range of the received backscatter signal strength needs to be compressed to accommodate the grayscale display. This is done by amplifying the weak signal selectively. The higher the dynamic range, the finer the image; the lower the dynamic range, the coarser the image. This can increase the significance of the echo difference.
4. Gain: When the gain values are increased, the received signal is amplified. However, the sound output cannot be changed. Too much gain can cause noise. When 2D gain and output increase and frequency decreases, the penetration improves.
5. Time gain compensation: Time gain compensation is also called distance gain compensation. During propagation of the ultrasound wave through the tissue, the attenuation gradually increases, the degree of attenuation is increased by each centimeter per 1 dB, and the frequency of each megahertz is attenuated by 1 dB. Human body tissue acts as a filter and can make the difference between the near-field and far-field echo signal strength become up to 100 dB or more. To obtain a uniform image, the near-field and far-field echo signals can be suppressed and enhanced, respectively, to optimize the imaging.

The above keys are usually used to optimize the 2D images. For neonatal lung scanning, we seldom use the color mode. We use the color mode to distinguish the vessels from branches filled with water. Due to the movement and breaths of neonates, there is more color noise when the color mode is applied. Thus, we need to optimize the PRF (pulse repeat frequency), wall filter, and color gain to produce color only in the vessels.

1.3 Examination Method of Lung Ultrasound

1.3.1 Selection of the Transducer

A linear transducer is used in neonate lung ultrasound and for premature infants. A high-frequency linear transducer can provide a high resolution. If there is a matrix linear probe, the elevational resolution will be better than that of the traditional probe.

In the absence of a suitable linear transducer, the use of a convex array transducer can be considered, but the highest frequency should be selected as much as possible.

1.3.2 Examination Method

Usually, with anterior and posterior axillary lines as the borders, the lungs are divided into three regions: anterior, lateral, and posterior regions. The two lungs are divided into six regions.

When ultrasound examination is performed on the lungs, it is necessary to perform longitudinal (the transducer is vertical to the ribs) or transverse (the transducer runs along the intercostal space) scans on each region of the lungs, and the longitudinal scan (parallel to the body longitudinal axis) is the most important and most common.

1.3.3 Precautions in Ultrasound Examination

1. The examiners should be skilled in the operating techniques.
2. Follow the routine operating procedures of the instrument to operate.
3. Try to minimize adverse stimulation on the newborns. The examination is usually carried out bedside, especially for high-risk children. The coupling agent should be preheated and kept warm to reduce heat loss. The examinations should be carried out when the children are quiet; it would be best when the child is sleeping. Generally, sedatives should not be used unless there is a medical indication. If necessary, a small amount of 10% chloral hydrate enema or comfort nipples should be used.
4. Notice on disinfection and isolation: Operators should wash their hands no matter what part of the newborn is scanned. After complete examination, the transducer should be cleaned and disinfected to avoid cross infection. Upon the cleaning and disinfection of the transducer, the following procedures should be used as follows:
   (a) First, rinse with water or wipe contaminants on the transducers with a soft cloth; if the transducer surface has dry and hard contaminants that are not easily removed, you can use Enzol® enzyme cleaning agent to assist in the cleaning.
   (b) After the transducer is cleaned, T-Spray™ and T-Spray II™ are used for disinfection. T-Spray™ and T-Spray II™ do not contain alcohol and phenol and will not induce the transducer damages.
   (c) If the transducer is heavily polluted, after the transducer is cleaned, immerse it into Cidex Plus® (3.4% glutaraldehyde solution) for 20 min (high levels of bactericide) at 25 °C for effective disinfection. For more detailed information about transducer cleaning and disinfection, please refer to http://www.civco.com/.

Currently, a simpler and more time-saving method is to use a protective jacket. The protective jacket covers the transducer surface, and the partial transducer lines are in contact with the incubator. Then, the sterile coupling agent is sprayed for scanning. After the examination of each newborn is finished, the previous protective jacket is replaced with a new one.

References

1. Weinberger SE, Drazen JM. Diagnostic procedures in respiratory diseases. In: Fuhlbrigge AL, Choi AMK, editors. Harrison's principle of internal medicine. 16th ed. New York: McGraw-Hill; 2005. p. 1505–8.
2. Desai SR, Hansel DM. Lung ultrasound in the adult respiratory distress syndrome: current practice and new insights. Intensive Care Med. 1997;23:7–15.
3. Lichtenstein DA. Lung ultrasound in the critically ill. Ann Intensive Care. 2014;4:1.
4. Wagner PR, Hedrick WR. Point-of-care ultrasound fundamental: principles, devices, and patient safety. 1st ed. New York: McGraw-Hill Education/Medical; 2014. p. 5–17.
5. Ziskin MC, Thickman DI, Goldenberg NJ, Lapayowker MS, Becker JM. The comet tail artifact. J Ultrasound Med. 1982;1(1):1–7.
6. Avruch L, Cooperberg PL. The ring-down artifact. J Ultrasound Med. 1985;4(1):21–8.
7. Louvet A, Bourgeois J. Lung ring-down artefact as a sign of pulmonary alveolar-interstitial disease. Vet Radiol Ultrasound. 2008;49(4):374–7.
8. Feldman MK, Katyal S, Blackwood MS. Ultrasound artifacts. Radiographics. 2009;29:1179–89.
9. Lee FCY. Lung ultrasound—a primary survey of the acutely dyspneic patient. J Intensive Care. 2016;4:57.

2 Sonographic Manifestations of Normal Lungs

Hai-Ying Cao and Erich Sorantin

2.1 Common Terms of Lung Ultrasound

The first step required to learn and master lung ultrasound is to become familiar with and understand the basic concepts and terminology that are at the basis of using ultrasound to diagnose lung diseases.

1. Pleural line [1, 2]: The echo reflection of the pleural is formed by interface of the pleural lung surface. The linear hyperechoic structure that manifests as smooth and regular under the ultrasound is called the pleural line (Fig. 2.1). Under normal circumstances, the disappearance, roughness, significant thickening, or irregularity of the pleural line represents an abnormality. There are two kinds of artifacts that stem from the pleural line. One is the horizontal A-line, and the other is perpendicular B-line. These two artifacts are perpendicular to each other and lay a foundation for lung ultrasound.
2. A-line [3]: The A-line is one kind of reverberation artifact located below the pleural line. It presents as a series of horizontal linear hyperechoic structures parallel to the pleural line; these are equidistant from each other and become weakened in echo strength with increasing depth, and the spacing is the distance from the skin to the pleural line. The number of A-lines is associated with the depth of the ultrasound machine; when the exploration position is relatively deeper, more A-lines are visibly displayed on screen.
3. B-line, comet-tail artifacts, and compact B-line [4, 5]: The B-line is one kind of laser-like vertical hyperechoic artifact that arises from the pleural line; it spreads to the edge of the screen without fading and synchronously moves with lung sliding and respiratory movements (Figs. 2.2, 2.3, and 2.4). We think whether the B-line reaches the edge of the screen or not depends on the setting of the depth. The B-line indicates filling of intralobular or interlobular septa, and it is invisible per intercostal in 30% of the lungs of normal children or adults under the ultrasound. However, as the lungs of newborns are rich in liquid, a small quantity of B-lines are visible on the ultrasound. There are two points to note here: (1) Previous findings in the literature indicate that B-lines and

Electronic Supplementary Material The online version of this chapter (https://doi.org/10.1007/978-94-024-1549-0_2) contains supplementary material, which is available to authorized users.

H.-Y. Cao (✉)
Department of Ultrasound, GE Healthcare, Beijing, China
e-mail: hai_ying.cao@china.med.ge.com

E. Sorantin
Division of Pediatric Radiology, Department of Radiology, Medical University Graz, Graz, Austria

J. Liu et al. (eds.), *Neonatal Lung Ultrasonography*, https://doi.org/10.1007/978-94-024-1549-0_2

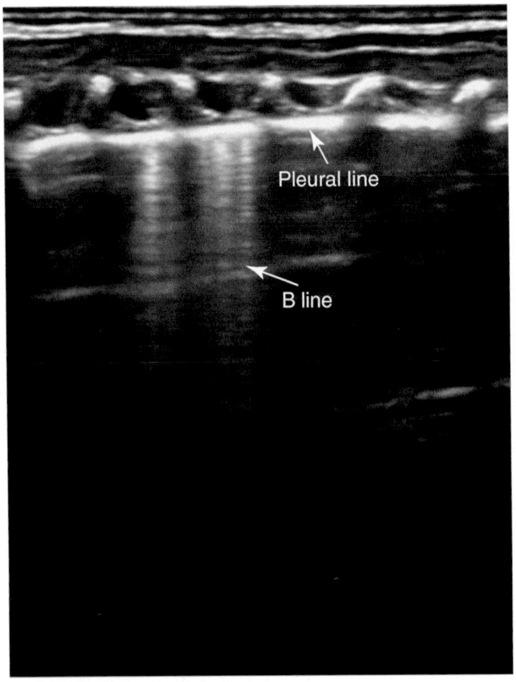

Fig. 2.1 Pleural line and B-line

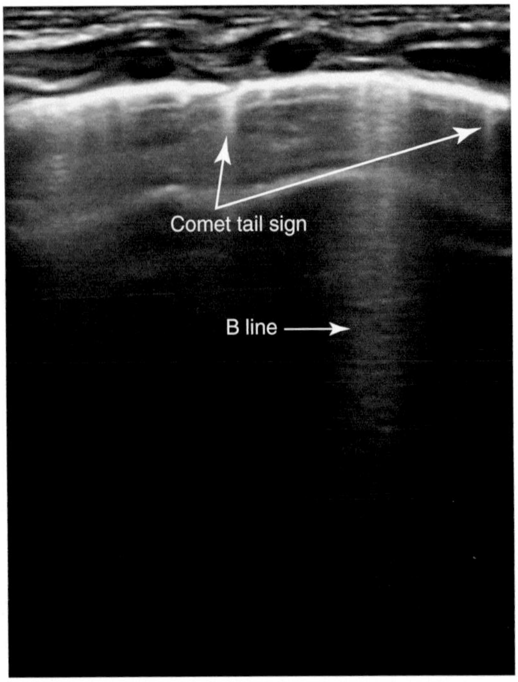

Fig. 2.2 B-line and comet-tail sign

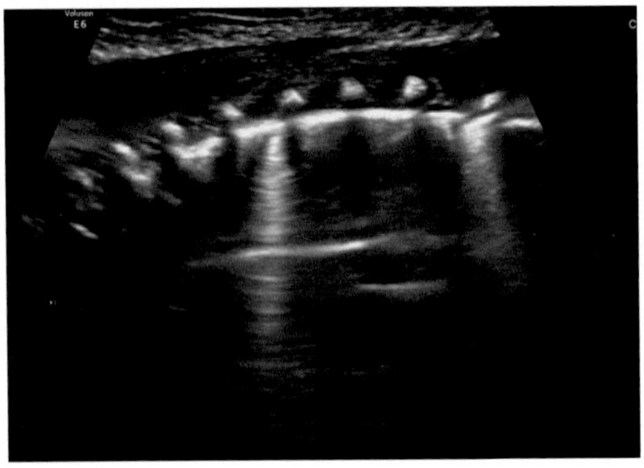

Fig. 2.3 B-line under real-time ultrasound (Video 2.1)

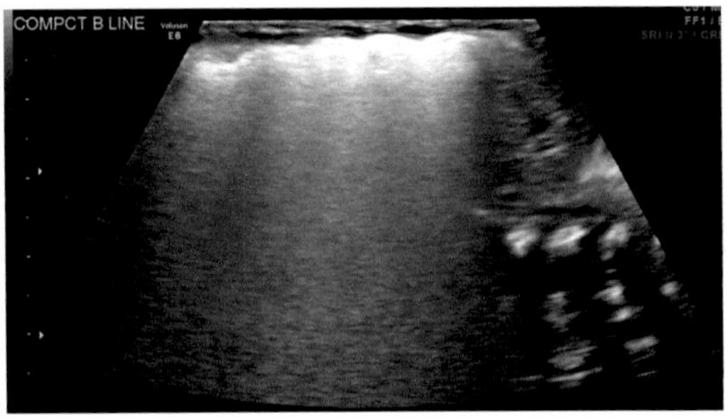

Fig. 2.4 Compact B-line. In compact B-line, the transducer is vertical to the ribs, no acoustical shadow of the ribs is displayed, and the entire lung field presents the dense B-line

comet-tail signs can completely disappear within 48–72 h after birth, but in our experience, a few lines or comet-tail signs can be present during the neonate period in small premature infants. (2) In the past, it has been considered that the A-line would disappear in the presence of B-lines; however, we find that after long-term clinical practice, B-lines and the A-line can coexist. This is not only seen early in disease and during disease recovery but is also found to a lesser extent of disease in children and part of the normal newborn. Compact B-lines refer to coalescent (dense) B-lines without rib shadows as a result of B-lines fused together (Fig. 2.5). Comet tails are short-path reverberation artifacts that weaken with each reverberation, resulting in vertical echogenic artifacts that rapidly fade as they continue further into the ultrasound image, resembling the shape of a comet tail.

4. Lung sliding [1]: During real-time ultrasound, it can be seen that the pleural line can move with the movement of respiration and

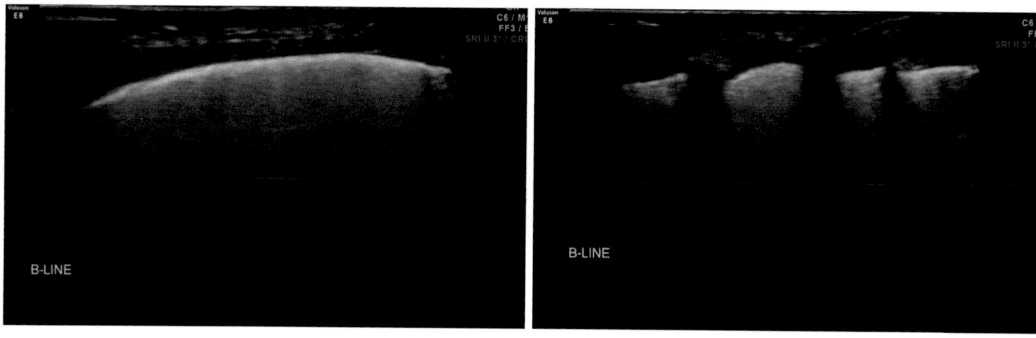

Fig. 2.5 The differentiation of compact B-line and B-line. The transducer is placed in the intercostal space, and the scan is performed when the transducer is parallel to the ribs. The in-field manifestation is similar to that of a compact B-line, but it is not actually the compact B-line (left diagram). When the scan is performed with the transducer rotating 90° to align vertically to the ribs, rib echoes are visible subcutaneously, as the field of vision is manifested as B-lines and ribs acoustic shadow, so these can be differentiated

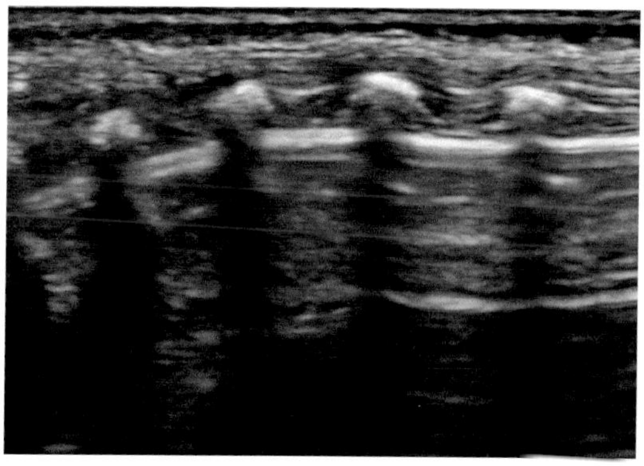

Fig. 2.6 Lung sliding (Video 2.2)

presents the relative movement of the chest wall of upper and lower round trip, which is called "lung sliding" (Fig. 2.6).

5. Lung consolidation [3, 6]: An ultrasonic image presents the lung tissues with "hepatization," probably associated with air bronchograms or fluid bronchograms. Lung consolidation is one of the most important signs in lung ultrasound imaging and is of vital value to the diagnosis of respiratory distress syndrome, pneumonia, and atelectasis (Figs. 2.7, 2.8, and 2.9).
6. Spared areas [2]: The normal lung tissues are surrounded by at least one intercostal area size and alveolar-interstitial syndrome (AIS) region (Fig. 2.10).
7. Alveolar-interstitial syndrome (AIS) [2]: When more than two B-lines are present in each the lung field, it is called alveolar-interstitial syndrome (Fig. 2.11).

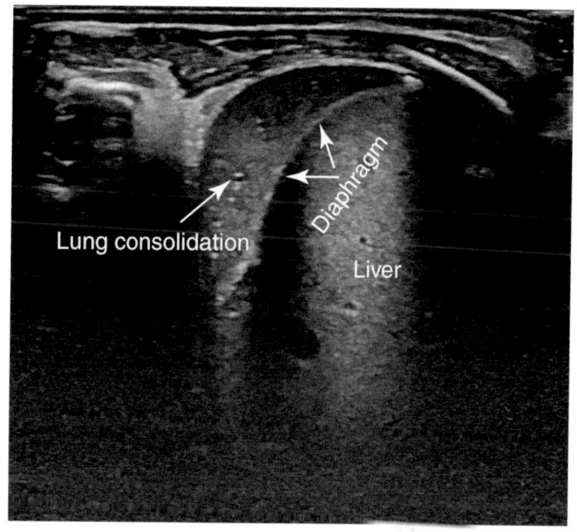

Fig. 2.7 Lung consolidation

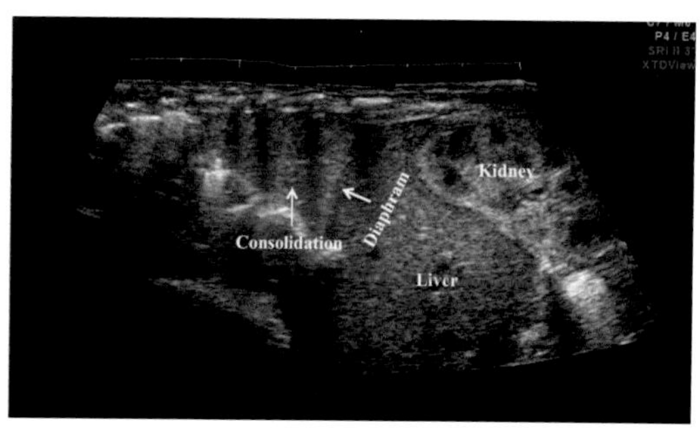

Fig. 2.8 Lung consolidation

8. Diffuse white lung [2]: The six regions of the lung field are manifested as dense B-lines, disappearance of A-lines, and no presence of "spared area." "White lung" is a

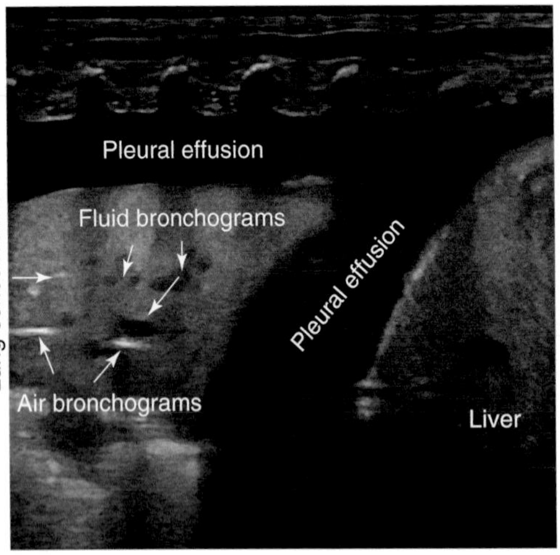

Fig. 2.9 Lung consolidation with air bronchograms and fluid bronchograms

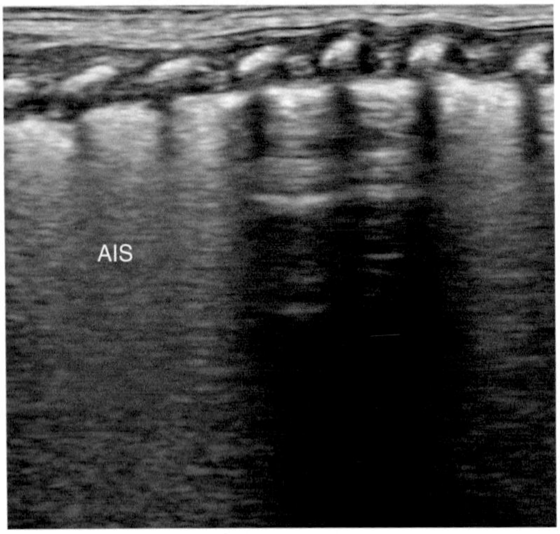

Fig. 2.10 Spared area

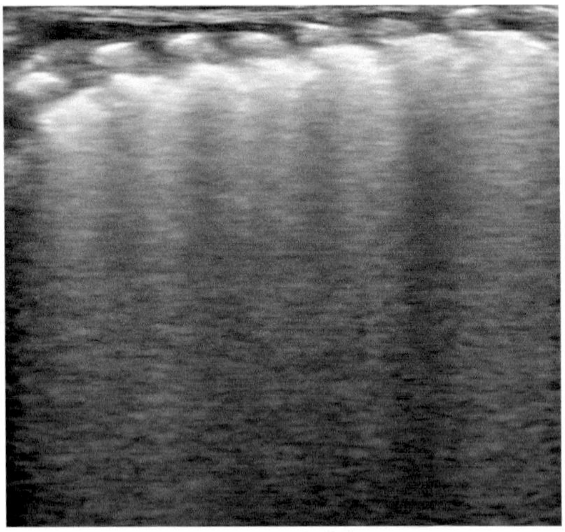

Fig. 2.11 Alveolar-interstitial syndrome

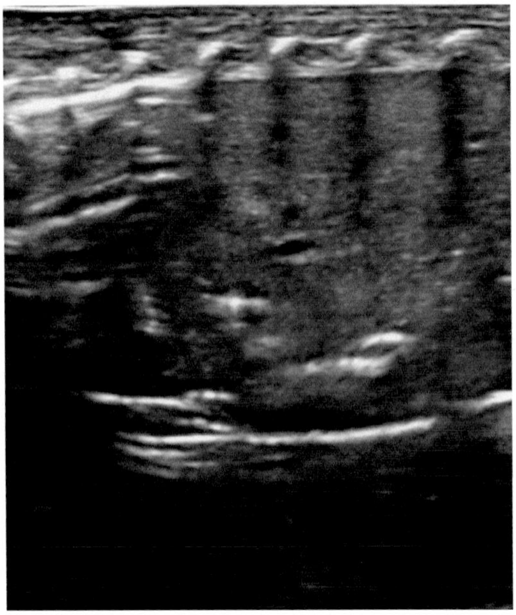

Fig. 2.12 Lung pulse (Video 2.3)

manifestation of serious AIS and is induced by the presence of a large amount of liquid in the pulmonary interstitium and alveoli.

9. Lung pulse [7]: The pulmonary tissues, with disappearance of lung sliding and visible consolidation at the pleural lines, beat with the heart pulsation. Lung pulsation is an important ultrasonic imaging characteristic of serious lung consolidation (such as atelectasis). Lung pulse can be observed and measured through the real-time two-dimensional ultrasound or M-mode (Figs. 2.12 and 2.13).
10. Lung point [8]: Under real-time ultrasound, the existence of a transition point with respiratory movement between the intermittent presence and absence of a lung sliding is called the lung point. The lung point is a specific sign of pneumothorax and can accurately locate the position of the gas boundary when mild-moderate pneumothorax is present.
11. Double lung point [9]: Due to differences in severity or the nature of pathological changes in different areas of the lung, a longitudinal scan shows a clear difference between upper and lower lung fields; this

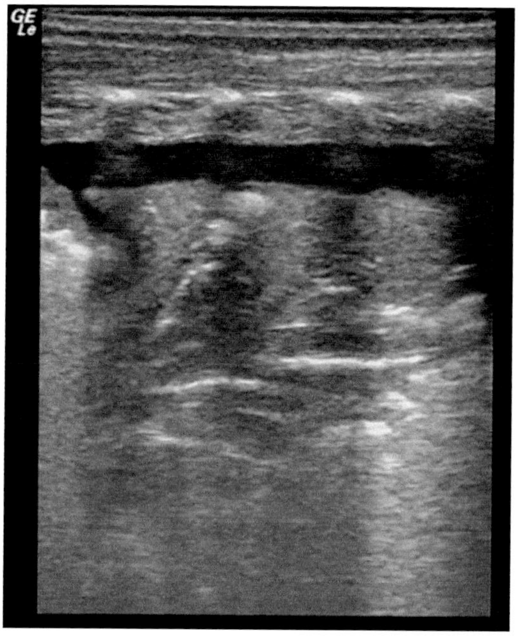

Fig. 2.13 Lung pulse (Video 2.4)

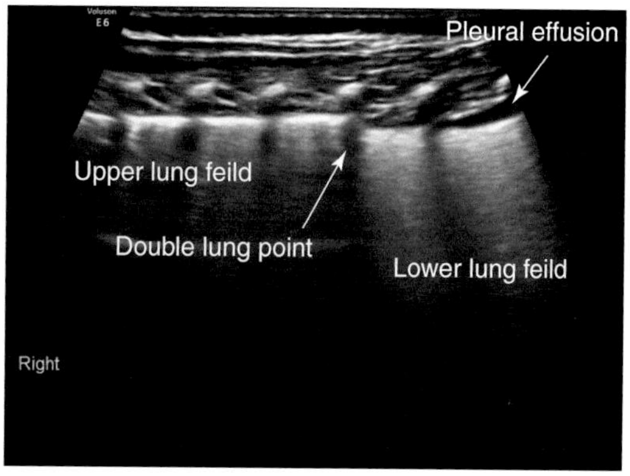

Fig. 2.14 Double lung point

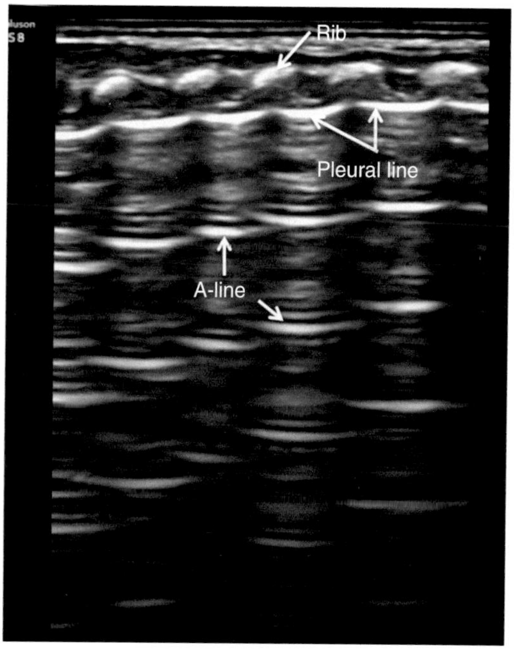

Fig. 2.15 Sonographic appearance of normal lungs of neonates

sharp cutoff point between the upper and lower lung field is known as a "double lung point" (Fig. 2.14).

12. Sandy beach sign and stratosphere sign [10, 11]: Under M-mode ultrasonography, a series of wavy line high echoes above the pleural line and the uniform granular dot echo (which is generated by lung sliding) below the pleural line can together form a beach-like sign known as a sandy beach or seashore sign. When lung sliding disappears, the granular dot echoes are replaced by a series of horizontal parallel lines, and this type of ultrasonic sign is known as a stratosphere or barcode sign.

2.2 Ultrasonic Image Characteristics of Normal Lungs of Neonates

2.2.1 Ultrasonic Image Characteristics of Normal Lungs of Neonates [12]

Normal lung tissues present the hypoechoic. When we scan the lung longitudinally under B-mode ultrasound, both the pleural line and A-line appear as smooth, clear, linear-hyperechoic parallel lines, equidistant from one another. The A-line intensity fades with the increase of lung depth. No B-lines or comet-tail artifacts exist in children or adults, but they can be observed in healthy neonates within 3–7 days after birth because fetal lungs are full of fluid. We should not find AIS, pleural effusion, or consolidations (Fig. 2.15) in the lungs of healthy neonates, either. Under M-mode scanning, the normal lung filled presents the beach sign (also known as "the granular sign") (Fig. 2.16).

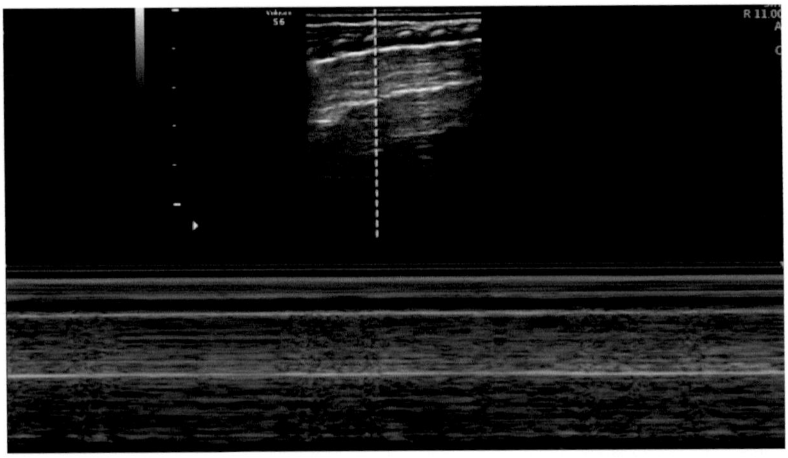

Fig. 2.16 Sonographic appearance of normal lungs in neonates under M-mode ultrasound, the lung fields appear as the beach sign

2.2.2 Indications of Lung Ultrasound Examinations [13]

The diagnosis of a variety of lung diseases, such as pneumothorax, pneumonia, atelectasis, pleural effusion, respiratory distress syndrome, pulmonary edema and interstitial syndrome, and alveolar-interstitial syndrome, as well as the recovery of diaphragmatic muscle abnormalities, dynamic observation of pneumonia and atelectasis, the ultrasound-guided retention of bronchoalveolar lavage liquid, and the suction of pleural effusion, is dependent upon lung ultrasound. This book will give an introduction to the ultrasound diagnosis of common lung diseases during the neonatal period.

2.2.3 Limitations of Lung Ultrasound

It is difficult for any technique to achieve perfection without the need for any modification, and lung ultrasound, which is still at the beginning stage of development, is no exception. Therefore, doctors need to pay attention to the limitations when using the lung ultrasound as a routine tool for the diagnosis of lung diseases. Scanning skill and the correct interpretation of images can be completed by operators who had been given formal training for a period of time and obtain necessary knowledge and skills. Several examinations need to be carried out every day so that the operators can become familiar with the skills and then they can master this technology and continue to explore it. In general, the diagnosis of pleural effusion, pulmonary consolidation, and alveolar-interstitial syndrome generally takes no more than 6 weeks. For diagnosis of pneumothorax and image capture, the operators need to go through long-term training, the main reason for which is the low incidence rate; in fact, pneumothorax image acquisition and diagnostic techniques are the hardest part of learning or training in lung ultrasound. Lung ultrasound also has its own inherent limitations, and this restriction does not depend on the operator but on the patient. As the fat layers of obese children are relatively thick, it is somewhat difficult to obtain good images. Subcutaneous emphysema also hinders the conduction of sound waves. Lastly and most importantly, ultrasound cannot be used for diagnosing emphysema.

References

1. Lichtenstein DA, Menu Y. A bedside ultrasound sign ruling out pneumothorax in the critically Ill: lung sliding. Chest. 1995;108:1345–8.
2. Copetti R, Cattarossi L, Macagno F, et al. Lung ultrasound in respiratory distress syndrome: a useful tool for early diagnosis. Neonatology. 2008;94:52–9.
3. Lichtenstein DA, Lascols N, Mezière G, et al. Ultrasound diagnosis of alveolar consolidation in the critically ill. Intensive Care Med. 2004;30:276–81.
4. Winfocus. 1st International consensus conference on pleura and lung ultrasound; 2010.

5. Marvin C, Ziskin MD, David I, et al. The comet tail artifact. J Ultrasound Med. 1982;1:1–7.
6. Volpicellia G, Silva F, Radeos M. Real-time lung ultrasound for the diagnosis of alveolar consolidation and interstitial syndrome in the emergency department. Eur J Emerg Med. 2010;17:63–72.
7. Lichtenstein DA, Lascols N, Prin S, Mezière G. The "lung pulse": an early ultrasound sign of complete atelectasis. Intensive Care Med. 2003;29(12):2187–92.
8. Piette E, Daoust R, Denault A. Basic concepts in the use of thoracic and lung ultrasound. Curr Opin Anaesthesiol. 2013;26(1):20–30.
9. Copetti R, Cattarossi L. The "double lung point": an ultrasound sign diagnostic of transient tachypnea of the newborn. Neonatology. 2007;91(3):203–9.
10. Lichtenstein D, Mezière G, Biderman P, Gepner A. The "lung point": an ultrasound sign specific to pneumothorax. Intensive Care Med. 2000;26(10):1434–40.
11. Lichtenstein DA, et al. Ultrasound diagnosis of occult pneumothorax. Crit Care Med. 2005;33(6):1231–8.
12. Liu J. Lung ultrasonography for the diagnosis of neonatal lung disease. J Matern Fetal Neonatal Med. 2014;27(8):856–61.
13. Volpicelli G, Elbarbary M, Blaivas M, et al. International evidence-based recommendations for point-of-care lung ultrasound. Intensive Care Med. 2012;38:577–91.

Neonatal Respiratory Distress Syndrome

3

Jing Liu and Erich Sorantin

Neonatal respiratory distress syndrome (NRDS), also known as hyaline membrane disease (HMD), refers to a severe lung disease with the main clinical manifestations of dyspnea, cyanosis, and respiratory failure in newborns shortly after birth. This disease results from the formation of additional eosinophilic hyaline membranes and pulmonary atelectasis from the alveolar wall to the terminal bronchiole wall caused by the primary or secondary absence of pulmonary surfactant (PS) due to various reasons. The disease was previously believed to occur mainly in premature infants; the younger the gestational age and the lower the weight of the infant at birth, the higher the incidence of this disease is. However, recently, with the conventional application of antenatal corticosteroids and/or PS prevention in the delivery room as well as the early development of INSURE (intubation-surfactant-extubation) technology, severe and typical respiratory distress syndrome (RDS) has become increasingly rare in preterm infants, while there have been more and more reports of full-term infants with RDS. RDS is one of the main causes of neonatal respiratory problems and death; therefore, more attention has been paid to this disease by neonatologists and obstetricians.

3.1 Respiratory Distress Syndrome in Premature Newborn Infants

3.1.1 Incidence

The incidence of RDS in premature infants is closely related to the gestational age and the birth weight. The younger the gestational age and the lower the weight of the infant at birth, the higher the incidence of this disease. For example, the incidence in infants at a gestational age less than 28 weeks is 80%; for those at 29 weeks, 60%; for those at 32–34 weeks, 15–30%; for those at 35–37 weeks, 5%; and for those at 39 weeks, almost 0%. The incidence in infants with a birth weight below 750 g is 80%; for those with a birth weight of 750–1000 g, it is 55% [1].

3.1.2 Etiology and Pathogenesis

1. Absence of pulmonary surfactant: Pulmonary surfactant (PS) is a phospholipid-protein complex that is synthesized and secreted by alveolar type II epithelial cells. It covers the alveolar surface, lowers the alveolar surface tension, maintains the functional residual capacity,

J. Liu (✉)
Department of Neonatology and NICU, Beijing Chaoyang District Maternal and Child Health Care Hospital, Beijing, China

E. Sorantin
Division of Pediatric Radiology, Department of Radiology, Medical University Graz, Graz, Austria

J. Liu et al. (eds.), *Neonatal Lung Ultrasonography*, https://doi.org/10.1007/978-94-024-1549-0_3

reduces exudate of liquid from the capillaries to the alveolae, stabilizes alveolar pressure, and prevents expiratory alveolar collapse. In the absence of PS, the alveolar surface tension increases. According to the formula P (alveolar retraction) = $2T$ (surface tension)/r (radius of alveolar), the small radius of the alveoli during end-expiration collapses first, and then pulmonary atelectasis occurs. Phosphatides account for 80–85% of PS, in which phosphatidylcholine (i.e., lecithin/phosphatidylcholine, PC, which is also known as lecithin) is the most important substance that functions as surfactant. It is produced during pregnancy beginning at approximately 18–20 weeks and increases slowly, and then production rises rapidly at approximately 35–36 weeks; thus, preterm infants born before 37 weeks lack such substances. Phosphatidylglycerol (PG) and sphingomyelin come next. PG has the lowest concentration before 26–30 weeks, increases along with PC after 30 weeks, reaches its peak at 36 weeks, and then declines to 1/2 the peak at full term (40 weeks). The sphingomyelin content remains relatively constant (there is only a small peak at 28–30 weeks); therefore, the L/S (lecithin/sphingomyelin) ratio in amniotic fluid or tracheal secretions is usually used to determine the maturity of the lungs. Protein accounts for 10–13% of PS, and approximately 50% of this protein can bind to PS and is called surfactant protein (SP). This binding with phospholipid can enhance surfactant production, including SP-A, SP-B, SP-C, and SP-D.

2. Hyperinsulinism (increased plasma insulin level): In the fetus, plasma adrenal cortical hormones can promote the synthesis of PS, while insulin can inhibit PS synthesis by adrenal cortical hormones. Therefore, if the fetal plasma insulin level increases, it will inhibit the synthesis of PS, which is detrimental to lung maturation. This is most common in infants with diabetic mothers, whose RDS incidence is five to six times higher than normal.
3. Formation of α_1-antitrypsin: α_1-antitrypsin (1-AT) is involved in the formation of the pulmonary hyaline membrane. α_1-AT can inhibit a variety of cathepsins and plays an important role in maintaining the structure and function of the lung. The formation of the pulmonary hyaline membrane may be due to plasminogen activator deficiency, while α_1-AT suppresses the profibrinolytic effect, which prevents plasma fibrin exudation from being degraded by plasmin, resulting in the formation of the pulmonary hyaline membrane.

3.1.3 Pathophysiological Changes

Previously, NRDS was called HMD based on specific pathological changes. Histological examination could detect adverse alveolar changes. The absence of alveolar surfactant and increases in alveolar surface tension (i.e., alveolar retraction force) cause the alveolus with the minimum radius to collapse, ultimately resulting in pulmonary atelectasis, pulmonary hypoventilation, decreased tidal volume, and decreased alveolar ventilation volume. However, normal pulmonary blood flow and a reduced lung ventilation/perfusion ratio cause metabolic acidosis and mixed acidosis, thereby resulting in increased pulmonary arterial spasm, pulmonary artery pressure and pulmonary vascular resistance, a foramen ovale, and a patent ductus arteriosus, which ultimately lead to a right-to-left shunt and persistent fetal circulation. Decreased pulmonary perfusion and exacerbation of lung tissue hypoxia result in increased permeability of the alveolar walls and alveolar capillaries, while fluid exudation, pulmonary interstitial edema, and exudation of fibrin are deposited at the alveolar surface and lead to the formation of an eosinophilic hyaline membrane, thus aggravating the gas diffusion barriers and hypoxic acid poisoning, which further inhibits PS synthesis and forms a vicious cycle.

3.1.4 Clinical Manifestations

Whether the baby is healthy or suffering from asphyxia at birth, shortly after birth (within 6 h, and for most infants within 1–3 h), the baby develops into progressive dyspnea, which reaches the most severe at 12–72 h. The manifestations are shortness of breath, cyanosis, retractions, and flaring nares, grunting, and later irregular breathing with occasional apnea. An expiratory groan is a protective reaction of the body, when the glottis is not fully open, to retain a small amount of gas in the lungs to prevent the alveolae from collapsing.

Almost all cases present with these symptoms within 12 h, and in cases in which symptoms present after 12 h, the signs are generally not due to hyaline membrane disease. Lung auscultation reveals decreased lung sounds or fine rales and hypotonia, systemic edema, and poor terminal circulation, and oliguria also occurs. Early heart sounds are still powerful but are weakened later, with bradycardia and low blood pressure (relatively high pulmonary artery pressure). After the second day, grades II–III systolic murmurs can be heard at the left sternal border or at the base of the heart (rarely heard on the first day).

The younger the gestational age and the lower the birth weight, the higher the incidence of this disease is. The incidence of RDS in infants with diabetic mothers is five to six times higher than that in those with normal mothers. PS synthesis is subject to the body fluid pH value, body temperature, and pulmonary blood flow. Therefore, the fetal blood volume changes caused by perinatal asphyxia, low temperature, placenta previa, placental abruption, and maternal hypotension will lead to the occurrence of RDS. The incidence of RDS is also higher in infants born by cesarean section, in second babies, and in boys born as twins.

3.1.5 Examination

1. Fluorescent tests: Within 30 min after birth, take 1 mL gastric juice and place it in a test tube with 1 mL of 95% ethyl alcohol. Shake hard for 15 s, and let it stand for 15 min. Then, observe the foam in the tube. The presence of PS promotes the formation and stability of foam, while ethyl alcohol has an inhibitory effect, and as a result, the amount of foam is the basis for a preliminary diagnosis of RDS. A (−) result means no foam and supports hyaline membrane disease; a (±) result is associated with a tiny amount of foam in the peripheral surface of the test tube and is suspicious for HMD; a (+) result indicates double layers or multiple layers of foam and rules out hyaline membrane disease, and this shows the presence of sufficient surfactant.
2. PS determination: Take amniotic fluid or tracheal fluid or tracheal aspirates from the infant to determine the *L*/*S* ratio. When the *L*/*S* is greater than or equal to 2, it indicates "lung maturity"; when the *L*/*S* is smaller than 1.5, it shows "immaturity of lungs." When the ratio is in between these values, it is suspicious for HMD.
3. Analysis of arterial blood gas: This test can reveal a respiratory or mixed acidosis, hypoxia, and hypercapnia.
4. Electrolyte and blood glucose disorders: The serum sodium level is decreased, but the serum potassium level remains normal in the early stages and may increase in the late stages. The serum calcium level usually decreases significantly after 72 h; and the blood glucose level also decreases.
5. Lung X-ray manifestations: This is an important clinical diagnosis method with a reliability as high as 80–85%, and it can be performed within 24 h after birth. Poor lung inflation, reduced brightness of the lung fields bilaterally, alveolar collapse forming granular or small nodular opacities, and alveolar ducts and terminal bronchioles with inflatable expansion forming reticular shadows can be seen, and lesions can be limited to one side or one lobe. As the upper lobe matures earlier than the lower lobe, the lower lobe has more lesions and more serious lesions. Typical fea tures can be seen 3–4 h after birth.
   (a) Bronchial inflatable sign: Due to widespread alveolar collapse, large amounts of gas accumulate in the airway, radiating outward to the terminal airways from the hilum, similar to the individual bifurcating branches.
   (b) Good thoracic expansion and a normal transverse septum: With excessive

expansion the alveolar ducts and the terminal bronchioles are enough to replace the capacity of the atrophic alveolae, thus causing thoracic expansion. The cardiothoracic ratio can be increased from 5 to 10% in the acute stages, and signs of pulmonary edema may appear. Based on the disease progress, the X-ray changes can be divided into four phases: Phase I (early phase), a shadow of fine mesh particles with a uniform distribution; Phase II, air bronchograms appear, over the cardiac silhouette, with consolidation in both lungs; Phase III, the lesion is further aggravated, with a ground-glass appearance and indistinct cardiac silhouette; and Phase IV (advanced phase), the density of the lung field is generally increased, and the cardiac silhouette disappears, which is known as the "white lung."

3.1.6 Treatment

This disease is a self-limiting disease, with a natural course of approximately 5 days. After 72 h, newborns can generate a considerable amount of surfactant, and the lesions gradually resolve. Therefore, early diagnosis and early treatment are necessary. Treatment focuses on supplemental oxygen and improving pulmonary ventilation. In recent years, due to the application of mechanical ventilation and administration of pulmonary surfactant, the prognosis has greatly improved, and mortality has decreased significantly.

1. General treatment
   (a) Maintain a neutral temperature environment, and keep the abdominal wall temperature at 36.5 °C to reduce oxygen consumption. Keep the relative humidity >50%.
   (b) Monitor blood gas and keep the arterial partial pressure of oxygen at 50–80 mmHg. For respiratory acidosis, the major strategy should be improving patients' ventilation by metabolic acidosis. Sodium bicarbonate should be used for correction, and the pH value should be kept at more than 7.3. Sodium bicarbonate cannot only correct acidosis but also expand the pulmonary blood vessels, improve perfusion of the lung, and increase hemoglobin oxygen-carrying capacity. It can also be used while monitoring blood gases.
   (c) Monitor breathing, heart rate, blood pressure, and respiration to prevent cerebral edema and heart failure. In cases of heart failure, quick digitalis should be used. In cases of patent ductus arteriosus, indomethacin and ibuprofen can be used to close it. For serious cases, surgical ligation may be needed.
   (d) Use antibiotics to prevent or control infection and abide strictly by a system of disinfection and isolation.
   (e) Maintain nutrition and fluid and electrolyte balance. For patients with severe illness and an oxygen requirement >40%, in general, do not feed these patients by mouth. According to the patient's daily nutritional requirements, supply 1/5–1/6 of the requirements as liquid. On the first day, give 5–10% GS at 60–80 mL/kg and then gradually increase to 120–150 mL/(kg.day). Then, 2–3 days after birth, supply electrolyte solution with Na^+ 2–3 mmol/kg and K^+ 1–2 mmol/kg. For patients with a caloric deficiency, consider intravenous hyperalimentation.
2. Oxygen therapy and assisted respiration
   (a) Mild (X-ray grade I): A nasal cannula, mask, or head cover can be used to administer oxygen inhalation by atomization, maintaining PaO_2 of 50–80 mmHg and a $TcSO_2$ of 90–95%.
   (b) Moderate (X-ray grade II): Continuous positive airway pressure (CPAP) can be used. On the one hand, alveolar collapse requires some pressure for alveolar expansion to improve oxygenation and reduce intrapulmonary shunting; on the other hand, the early application of CPAP can maintain surfactant production, decrease

the demands for oxygen, reduce pulmonary complications, and improve the prognosis. The indications for the use of CPAP are as follows: (1) when the oxygen concentration is >60%, PaO_2 <6.7 kPa (50 mmHg), or $TcSO_2$ <85%, (2) apnea or cardiac arrhythmias, and (3) before withdrawing the ventilator, when the CPAP pressure is usually 4–6 (<10) cmH_2O (0.39–0.59 kPa), the gas flow rate is usually three times the amount of ventilation (6–8 mL/kg × respiratory rate × 3), which is usually 5–7 L/min, the temperature is 32 °C, and the humidity is 100%.

(c) Severe (X-ray grade III and over): Severe RDS tends to need conventional mechanical ventilation (CMV). The presence of one of the following indications should be treated with CMV: (1) CPAP pressure is ≥8 cmH_2O (0.78 kPa) with FiO_2 at 0.8, PaO_2 <6.7 kPa (50 mmHg), or $TcSO_2$ <85%; (2) $PaCO_2$ >70 mmHg (9.3 kPa) and pH <7.25; (3) frequent apnea or when CPAP, artificial stimuli, or drugs are ineffective; and (4) infants of a young gestational age with an FiO_2 ≥0.6; for example, if PaO_2 <6.7 kPa (50 mmHg) or $TcSO_2$ <85%, CMV treatment should be directly administered. The general peak inspiratory pressure should be ≤30 cmH_2O (2.9 kPa), average airway pressure <10 cmH_2O (0.98 kPa), end-expiratory pressure 4–6 cmH_2O (0.39–0.59 kPa), respiratory rate 35–45 breaths/min, and inspiration/expiration ratio = 1:1–2.

(d) High-frequency ventilation (HFV): Conventional mechanical ventilation reduces the mortality of RDS but increases the risk of serious complications, such as bronchial pulmonary dysplasia, gas leakage, ventilator-associated pneumonia, retinopathy, intracranial hemorrhage, and persistent patent ductus arteriosus. In recent years, the use of a high-frequency positive pressure shock wave for ventilation and gas access to the respiratory tract with a 120–1200/min high-frequency oscillation waveform is an enhanced diffusion or forced diffusion ventilation method that lowers inspiratory pressure and reduces complications. However, the substitute for high-frequency ventilation in case of its invalidity is subject to personal experience, habits, and the nature of the lung disease.

3. Exogenous pulmonary surfactant replacement therapy

Administer the exogenous surfactant (natural or synthetic) through a tracheal cannula into the infant's trachea. First, remove the endotracheal secretions. Then, rotate the infant's position (such as from the supine position to the right lateral position, to the left lateral decubitus position, and again to the supine position). Administer a resuscitation capsule after each injection. Use positive pressure ventilation with the respirator for 1–2 min, with a uniform distribution. Between 20 min and 3 h after administration, there will be significant improvement in the blood gas analysis. After confirmation of the illness, the earlier the use of surfactant, the better the effect will be. Different PS preparations have different dosages and intervals (usually 6–12 h). Surfactant can be administered once or twice depending on the patient's situation, but should not exceed four administrations. After administering PS, the improvement in oxygenation in BPD is related to the dosage. Currently, the commonly used preparation in China is Curosurf (100–120 mg/kg each time) or Calsurf (70–100 mg/kg each time). Exogenous surfactant also has some side effects, for example, adverse effects on the hemodynamics of the systemic and pulmonary circulation, cardiac output, and cerebral perfusion. Thus, the application of exogenous surfactant may reduce infant mortality but leads to no significant improvement in intracranial hemorrhage, cerebral palsy, and neurobehavioral development.

4. Other therapies

Nitric oxide (NO) inhalation therapy is used for the treatment of pulmonary artery hypertension, especially in cases of persistent fetal circulation; conditions permitting, apply extracorporeal membrane oxygenation (ECMO), which is not currently well-developed.

3.1.7 Differential Diagnosis

1. Neonatal transient tachypnea (TTN): TTN, previously known as wet lungs, is due to an early neonatal pulmonary physiological function disorder and excess pulmonary fluid. The duration of symptoms is short with good prognosis. The general mechanism involves the following: (1) Imperfect function of the pulmonary lymphatic vessels and veins leads to retained fluid in the lung. (2) The inhalation of amniotic fluid leads to excessive fluid in the lungs. (3) A cesarean delivery does not allow the vaginal squeeze of the infant's chest. The clinical features of TTN include the following: (1) There are more full-term infants, cesarean infants, and perinatal infants, and the number of affected males is greater than that of females. (2) Shortness of breath occurs within 2–5 h after birth, with groaning or bruising, but no progressive aggravation of dyspnea, which disappears within 24 h. (3) There are few lung signs except decreased breath sound or coarse rales. (4) In most patients, a blood gas analysis is normal. (5) The treatment is mainly to strengthen the patient and provide symptomatic care. Lung X-rays mainly show the following: (1) The lung texture increases in thickness, similar to pulmonary congestion. (2) There is extensive patchy shading of the lung. (3) There is evidence of a leaf or/and pleural effusion. (4) These changes disappear mostly within 2–3 days.
2. Group B hemolytic streptococcal infection: Neonatal pneumonia and septicemia in the early stages can be caused by Group B hemolytic streptococcal intrauterine infections. The clinical manifestations and lung X-ray manifestations are very similar to pulmonary hyaline membrane disease, even involving hyaline membrane formation in the affected lung, which is not easily distinguished from hyaline membrane disease; however, the mother of a child with septicemia tends to have the history of sepsis or premature rupture of the fetal membranes for reference. A timely blood culture and the development of gastric juice or bronchial secretions within 12 h are helpful for diagnosis. In cases in which the infection is not easily identified, hyaline membrane disease may be diagnosed instead of a Group B hemolytic streptococcal infection.
3. Aspiration pneumonia or meconium aspiration syndrome: (1) born with a history of asphyxia or a history of meconium-stained amniotic fluid. (2) The affected area of the lung on X-ray is at the bottom of the lung without alveolar collapse or air bronchograms.
4. Atelectasis: This is a complication of a variety of lung diseases, and the main symptoms are intermittent cyanosis, respiratory irregularities and apnea, oxygen inhalation, or loss of bruising after crying or oxygen intake. Atelectasis appears as a patchy pattern or a dense shadow on X-rays. In cases of severe atelectasis, the heart and trachea may shift away from the diseased side.

3.1.8 Prevention

1. Prepare for pregnancy healthcare and prevent premature labor.
2. Prenatal maternal injection of corticosteroids: Inspect the amniotic fluid of pregnant women with the possibility of premature labor, and administer adrenal cortical hormones 24–48 h before delivery (domestic commonly used dexamethasone, 10 mg/day × 1–2 days).
3. Prenatal maternal injection of a large dose of ambroxol hydrochloride: The injection of a large-dose ambroxol hydrochloride to pregnant women with the possibility of preterm delivery for 3–5 days before delivery can reduce the number of preterm infants with RDS and intracranial hemorrhage and infant mortality rates.
4. Injection of pulmonary surfactant into the amniotic cavity: Pulmonary surfactant in the amniotic fluid can enter the fetal lung by fetal breathing movements, so the injection of pulmonary surfactant into the amniotic cavity guided by prenatal ultrasound before delivery can prevent the occurrence of preterm infants

with RDS. The combination with a respiratory stimulant (such as aminophylline) may improve the curative effect.

5. For small gestational age and low birth weight infants, routinely give pulmonary surfactant after birth to significantly reduce the incidence of RDS and alleviate the severity of illness. In recent years, the application of artificial synthetic containing SP-B pulmonary surfactant (lucinactant) has received more significant attention abroad. Compared with conventional preparations, it can further reduce the incidence of RDS and decrease infant mortality of RDS-related BPD.

3.2 Respiratory Distress Syndrome in Full-Term Newborn Infants

In recent years, there have been more and more reports on full-term infants with RDS. Bouziri et al. have reported that 7% of near-term infants with RDS have acute respiratory distress syndrome (ARDS). Berthelot-Ricou et al. have reported that cesarean section delivery at 36 weeks and 37 weeks was associated with hospitalization due to severe RDS in 9.4% and 6.3% of infants, respectively. The Children's Hospital affiliated with Zhejiang University reported 177 cases with RDS, and 74 cases were late preterm or full-term infants, accounting for 42% of cases, which is almost half. In our full-term neonatal intensive care unit, RDS infants account for more than 3.6% of all hospitalized neonates [2–6]. Thus, RDS is not uncommon in full-term infants. However, the etiology and pathogenesis, clinical characteristics, and diagnosis and treatment of premature infants with RDS are significantly different from those of premature infants, which will be introduced.

3.2.1 Etiology, Classification, and Pathogenesis [5, 6]

The fundamental reason for RDS in premature infants is a deficiency in primary pulmonary surfactant, which is significantly different from full-term infants. According to our study results, the main risk factors for full-term infants with RDS include premature rupture of the fetal membranes, severe intrauterine infection, elective cesarean section, severe birth asphyxia, low birth weight, diabetes, and pregnancy tolerance abnormalities, and male sex. In addition, hereditary pulmonary surfactant deficiency is rare, but it is the main reason for full-term infants to have lethal RDS. According to the differences in etiology and pathogenesis, RDS in full-term infants is divided into three categories.

1. Idiopathic respiratory distress syndrome (IRDS): This disease is mainly found in elective cesarean delivery (ECD) infants with a gestational age ≤38, male infants, and infants born to diabetic mothers. The mechanism of RDS in infants born to diabetic mothers is relatively simple. It is associated with high concentrations of insulin in the blood that inhibit the promotion of antagonistic adrenocortical hormones on PS synthesis, which is a commonly known phenomenon. Here, we will mainly discuss the relationship between cesarean section and sex and RDS. (1) Association between elective cesarean section and RDS in full-term infants: ECD-related RDS is mainly found in full-term infants and late preterm infants. We have reported that in 125 cases of full-term infants RDS, nearly 30% have primary RDS, and ECD deliveries with a gestational age ≤38 weeks have a nearly 90% occurrence of RDS. Previous reports believed that the following factors led to the high incidence of RDS in ECD infants: (1) The low levels of endogenous glucocorticoids in ECD infants and catecholamines affect PS synthesis. Glucocorticoid levels in the neonatal cord blood should be determined before and after cesarean section delivery, and the latter should be five times the former. (2) Cesarean section delivery inhibits the removal of fetal lung fluid, and excessive fluid in the lungs results in decreased concentrations of PS in the lungs and decreased ventilation. During the fetal period, the regulation of Cl^- ion secretion in the fetal lung tissue accomplished by the airway epithelial cells produces enough lung fluid to maintain normal development of the

lung; at parturition and after birth, the lung fluid needs to be cleared rapidly in order to perform gas exchange. At present, it is believed that lung fluid clearance occurs by transfer through the alveolar epithelial cell membrane. These channels include Na^+ channels, K^+ channels, ATP-sensitive K^+ channel, Na^+-K^+-ATP enzymes, and aquaporin proteins (AQPs), of which the Na^+-K^+-ATP enzymes and the epithelial Na^+ channels (ENaCs) play major roles [12]. The basic process of lung fluid clearance occurs as follows:

(a) Cell membrane Na^+-K^+-ATP enzyme activation hyperpolarizes the basolateral membrane potential, which causes further increases in intracellular K^+ and extracellular Na^+, thus establishing a chemical concentration gradient for high intracellular K^+ and high extracellular Na^+.
(b) Intracellular K^+ reaches the extracellular space through basement membrane K^+ channels along a chemical gradient, resulting in a larger electrochemical gradient in cells, so that the Na^+ ion enters the lumen along a chemical gradient through apical membrane Na^+ channels.
(c) Na^+ absorption depolarizes the apical membrane potential, and Cl^- ions enter the lumen through Cl^- channels (cystic fibrosis transmembrane conductance regulator and cystic fibrosis transmembrane conduction regulatory protein, which are subject to cAMP regulation and are present in alveolar type I and type II epithelial cells).
(d) The movement of intracellular Na^+ and Cl^- ions forms an alveolar pulmonary interstitial osmotic gradient; thus, water molecules pass through cellular pathways and paracellularly from the alveolar space via epithelial cells and into the pulmonary interstitium and are cleared by the lymphatic system.
(e) The mechanical stimulation of vaginal delivery, sympathetic excitement due to the stress of birth, and increases in glucocorticoid and catecholamine secretion stimulate the activity of the Na^+-K^+-ATP enzyme and the ENaC, thereby increasing lung fluid clearance.

The abovementioned factors also exist in infants with a gestational age >38; however, after the gestational age exceeds 38 weeks, ECD significantly reduces the incidence of RDS. The abovementioned mechanisms are far from explaining the correlation between ECD and RDS. Therefore, it is believed that the ECD-induced iatrogenic preterm labor makes relatively small gestational age and the relative deficiency of PS the root cause of RDS incidence in these infants.

2. Gender relatedness to RDS in full-term infants: Gender and sex hormones are closely related to human health and disease, and it has been recognized that they are closely related to cardiovascular disease, musculoskeletal diseases, and nervous system diseases. Recently, it has been found that gender is related to many pulmonary diseases, such as allergic asthma, chronic obstructive pulmonary disease, pulmonary fibrosis, pulmonary hypertension, pulmonary fibrosis, and lung cancer. Our clinical study showed that three times more male full-term infants were affected by RDS than females (95%CI = 1.721–4.053). Multiple sex hormone receptors are present in the alveolar epithelial cell membrane, including three kinds of estrogen receptors (ER-α, ER-β, and GPER1), two kinds of progesterone receptors (PR-A and PR-B), and one androgen receptor (AR). Sex hormones regulate lung development and pulmonary function of mature infants by binding with their corresponding receptors, but different sex hormones produce different effects: (1) Androgens promote secretion of fibroblast-pneumonocyte factor (FPF) and, by delaying lung fibroblasts, delay the maturation of alveolar type II cells and reduce the release of PS. (2) Androgens affect the development of the lung by regulating the signal transduction pathway of epidermal growth factor (EGF) and transforming growth factor beta (TGF-β). (3) Estrogens can promote PS synthesis by affecting various components of PS, including phospholipids, lecithin, and lung surfactant

protein-A and protein-B (SP-A, SP-B). Estrogens can also promote the development of fetal lung maturity by increasing the number of alveolar type II cells and the formation of lamellar bodies. Therefore, compared with male infants with the same lung volume, the lungs of females develop and mature earlier in their anatomical and physiological features, including earlier development of the bronchial smooth muscle, earlier development of the terminal lung, faster increases in lung volume, earlier development of alveolar type I and type II epithelial cells, earlier production of PS, lower airway resistance, higher maximum expiratory flow rate, higher forced expiratory flow rate, and larger gas channels. (4) Bronchial smooth muscle is affected differently by different sex hormones, and estrogen may play a role in bronchiectasia through the following mechanisms: (a) Intracellular Ca^{2+} concentrations are reduced. This enhances K^+ channel activity and decreases cell membrane potential, thereby reducing voltage-dependent calcium channel activity. It also inhibits L-type Ca^{2+} channels, namely, the activity of store-operated calcium channels. The lowered intracellular Ca^{2+} concentrations and decreased intracellular Ca^{2+} release lead to bronchial smooth muscle relaxation. (b) Endogenous NO synthesis is stimulated and released via the PI3K-Akt-NO pathway. The binding of estrogen and GPER1 may activate phosphatidylinositol 3-kinase (PI3) that then further activates protein kinase B (Akt), enhancing the activity of endogenous nitric oxide synthase (eNOS), increasing NO production, and causing bronchodilation. (c) Estrogen can significantly enhance bronchial dilation via isopropyl noradrenaline.

3. Acute respiratory distress syndrome (ARDS, namely, RDS): At present, it is believed that ARDS is a kind of direct or indirect lung injury caused by nonspecific inflammatory reactions due to various pathogenic factors, accounting for the vast majority of RDS in full-term infants. Among the 125 full-term infants with RDS in our report, over 70% were infants with ARDS. The main reasons for developing ARDS include premature rupture of the fetal membranes, intrauterine infections (severe pneumonia and sepsis), severe asphyxia, meconium aspiration syndrome, pulmonary hemorrhage, and low birth weight.

   Premature rupture of the fetal membranes in full-term infants with RDS: Premature rupture of the fetal membranes is closely related to RDS, and several mechanisms are involved. (1) Premature or relative delivery can occur following premature rupture of the fetal membranes. (2) Decreased amniotic fluid can lead to RDS for several reasons. (a) Oligohydramnios may decrease the lung fluid due to external extrusion of the fetal thorax, and the fetal lung liquid content is equivalent to postnatal lung residual volume. Therefore, significantly reduced lung fluid will cause serious adverse effects on lung development. (b) The normal alveolar amniotic fluid pressure gradient plays an important role in maintaining fetal lung development, and a significant reduction in the amount of amniotic fluid and reduced amniotic fluid pressure result in lower alveolar amniotic fluid pressure gradient, which is another important reason for fetal pulmonary hypoplasia. (c) Oligohydramnios also limits the exchange of lung fluid and amniotic fluid, and some components in the amniotic fluid can stimulate the development of the lung. (d) Plenty of amniotic fluid volume can maintain mechanical compression of the fetal chest wall and maintain a normal pressure gradient in the respiratory tract, which is conducive to lung development. Furthermore, significant decreases in the quantity of amniotic fluid will limit the movement of the fetus, thorax and fetal lung, to some extent affecting the normal development of the lung. Oligohydramnios produces a significant adverse effect on fetal lung development in premature infants, while it does not generate a dominant effect on full-term infants. (3) Intrauterine infections and inflammation are related to preterm rupture of the fetal membranes. Influenced by infection and the inflammatory response and inflammatory factors, the fetal pulmonary microvascular integrity is damaged, the pulmonary capillary permeability increases, and large amounts of albumin exudate appear in the lung tissue, resulting in increased liquid content in the fetal lung, and lung tissues collapse, which causes reduced PS synthesis, increased damage, and reduced activity.

Severe (intrauterine) infections, severe asphyxia, meconium aspiration, and pulmonary hemorrhage and are all high-risk factors for full-term infants with RDS, and the possible mechanisms involve the following:

(a) Direct damage to alveolar type II cells.
(b) Aggregation of a large number of inflammatory cells and the release of inflammatory cytokines, leading to diffuse alveolar damage by mediating an inflammatory reaction.
(c) Inhibition of PS synthesis and damage to PS function caused by hypoxia and acidosis.
(d) Increased alveolar capillary permeability and destruction and inactivation of PS by plasma proteins and other ingredients that have gained access to the alveolae, resulting in severe non-cardiogenic pulmonary edema.
(e) Inactivation of PS following pulmonary hemorrhage by some of the ingredients in the blood, such as hemoglobin and red blood cells.
(f) Direct damage to the lung tissue by the cholate in the meconium-stained amniotic fluid.
(g) Dilution of PS caused by amniotic fluid inhalation that increases the lung fluid.
(h) Increased PS consumption due to disease progression when infants need greater amounts of PS.

4. Hereditary surfactant deficiency respiratory distress syndrome: Though hereditary PS deficiency is rare, it is related to multiple severe lung diseases. There have been reports on the relationship between the hereditary deficiency of four SP gradients (SP-A, SP-B, SP-C, and SP-D) and lung diseases, and hereditary PS deficiency is also the main reason for full-term lethal RDS. The most common hereditary SP deficiency that leads to RDS is caused by an SP-B gene mutation that is autosomal recessive. The most common variant is a frameshift mutation, in which GAA replaces C in the 121 codon position, namely, in the No. 4 of the 121 codon position of the SP-B gene, a pure 2 bp fragment (121ins2) is inserted, resulting in a premature termination codon (the estimated population carrying rate is 1 per thousand) and creating an obstacle for downstream codon encoding. Further studies have also found that the SP-B mutant gene can be normally transcribed but cannot produce stable mRNA and SP-B proteins, and the formation of SP-C is also blocked. According to estimates, RDS due to a hereditary SP-B deficiency accounts for 25% of refractory RDS in full-term infants. An ATP-binding cassette transporter A3 (ABCA3) gene mutation is one of the rare reasons for RDS caused by a hereditary SP deficiency. ABCA3 is a membrane-binding protein with a high molecular weight that exists widely in alveolar type II cells, has phospholipid surface activity, and participates in the formation of the lamellar plate. ABCA3 gene mutations not only cause ABCA3 deficiency but also result in abnormal treatment of SP-C and SP-B and abnormal metabolic pathways, thus leading to serious abnormalities in PS and RDS.

3.2.2 Clinical Features [5, 6]

According to our clinical observations, RDS in full-term infants has the following characteristics:

1. Secondary RDS (i.e., ARDS) is common, accounting for over 70% of cases; primary RDS accounts for less than 30%.
2. Severe infections (intrauterine infections, pneumonia, or sepsis) are the most common of ARDS in full-term infants.
3. The main cause for primary RDS is an elective cesarean section; the gender of the infant is the next cause. The chance of a boy suffering from RDS is three times greater than the chances of a girl.

4. The early onset of severe, rapidly progressing illness. Over 70% develop the disease within 3 h after birth; over 90%, within 6 h; and over 99%, within 12 h.

   However, some infants develop disease at a later time. Recently, we have identified one case. The infant developed severe asphyxia at birth (the Apgar score was less than 3 at 1, 5, and 10 min after birth). At admission an X-ray detected no obvious abnormalities. The patient was supported with conventional mechanical ventilation for central respiratory failure. At 36 h after birth, the infant presented with a sudden oxygen saturation decline and severe cyanosis. Frequent ventilation (PIP 30 cmH_2O, PEEP 5 cmH_2O, FiO_2 1.0, and RR 50 breaths/min), high-frequency ventilation (MAP >22 cmH_2O), and NO inhalational therapy could not relieve the cyanosis. Then, after immediately reviewing the X-ray examination, it showed grade IV RDS changes in the lungs
5. RDS in full-term infants can easily lead to sustained fetal circulation and multiple organ failure. Nearly 40% of infants suffer from multiple organ failure, and 20% have persistent fetal circulation (PFC)
6. The main cause of death is severe infection accompanied by multiple organ failure. The four cases of death we encountered all had multiple organ failure, including acute renal failure, severe myocardial injury (myocardial infarction and ventricular fibrillation), very severe acidosis (pH <6.8 and BE negative that could be detected), and persistent fetal circulation. The time of death in these cases was within 1 week after birth, but early and aggressive treatment can improve the prognosis.

Recently, some scholars have divided adult ARDS into three phases. Phase I or acute lung injury (ALI) involves acute onset dyspnea, pulmonary rales, extravascular lung water index (EVLWI) >7 mL/kg, oxygenation index <40 kPa, shunt volume 10–15%, and without left heart dysfunction. Phase II or RDS involves serious progressive dyspnea, diffuse lung wet rales, EVLWI beyond physical boundaries, oxygenation index <26.7 kPa, and a chest X-ray showing diffuse exudative lesions. In addition, Phase III is the terminal stage. According to the patient's prognosis, the outcome falls into three classes: (1) a good prognosis for pulmonary function recovery, (2) a decline in the quality of life associated with the development of pulmonary fibrosis and chronic obstructive pulmonary disease, and (3) a poor prognosis associated with the occurrence of sepsis, multiple organ dysfunction, or even death. It is believed that this classification method may be helpful for guiding the treatment of ARDS and improving the prognosis.

3.2.3 Diagnosis [5, 6]

Although PS deficiency is the root cause of RDS, there is still a lack of a reliable method for detecting PS until now. Therefore, the diagnosis of RDS is still dependent on assessing the clinical manifestations, arterial blood gas analyses, and chest X-ray examinations. In 1994, the American-European Consensus Conference (AECC) developed diagnostic criteria for adult ARDS: (1) acute onset, (2) PaO_2/FiO_2 ratio ≤26.7 kPa, (3) no left atrial pressure detected by an echocardiogram, and (4) an X-ray examination showing no exudative lesions in either lung. In 1989, *Pediatrics* used the following criteria to describe RDS in full-term infants: (1) full-term newborns with acute onset; (2) perinatal inducing factors; (3) chest X-ray examination showing that both lungs were diffusely affected and decreased; (4) continuous positive pressure ventilation required for more than 48 h, with FiO_2 >0.5 for at least 12 h; (5) PEEP ≥6 cmH_2O over 3 days; and (6) dyspnea caused by other reasons. In 2007, *Tunis Med* used the following diagnostic criteria to describe RDS in full-term and near-term infants: (1) gestational age ≥35 weeks, (2) acute and severe breathing difficulties requiring conventional mechanical ventilation with PEEP ≥4 cmH_2O and FiO_2 = 0.5 for more than 6 h, (3) oxygen dependence for more than 48 h, (4) chest X-ray examination showing diffuse changes, and (5) a PaO_2 ≤60 mmHg when the inhaled oxygen concentration ≥0.5. Combining the relevant literature and clinical observations, we put forward the following criteria: (1) term newborns with acute onset; (2) clear perinatal trigger factors such as selective cesarean section, intrauterine infection, severe asphyxia, meconium aspiration, or pulmonary hemorrhage; (3) typical clinical manifestations including dyspnea occurring shortly after birth, grunting, retractions, cyanosis, and significantly reduced or absent breath sounds on lung auscultation; (4) typical RDS X-ray changes in the lung; (5) arterial blood gas analysis showing hypoxia and high blood $PaO_2/FiO_2 \leq 26.7$ kPa; and (6) exclusion of breathing difficulties caused by severe pneumonia, meconium aspiration, or pulmonary hemorrhage.

3.2.4 Treatment Strategies [5, 6]

1. Early and active conventional mechanical ventilation: RDS in full-term infants is mainly secondary and often progresses rapidly. When oxygen inhalation via a head mask or CPAP-assisted respiration is not needed, the oxygenation status is good because the compensatory ability of the infants at this time is good. Once oxygenation cannot be maintained and decompensates, the disease tends to be extremely critical. Conventional mechanical ventilation at this time becomes very difficult, and it is even hard to save the lives of the infants. Therefore, immediate administration of conventional mechanical ventilation after the diagnosis is confirmed is one of the important measures for successful treatment in full-term infants with RDS. Some specific notes include the following: (1) Remember not to perform "head cover/CPAP/conventional mechanical ventilation" treatment procedures. (2) It is usually necessary to have higher ventilation parameters, especially in terms of PIP and PEEP, and physicians should not be satisfied with fair oxygenation status of infants with lower parameters. Animal experiments have proved that, compared with lung-protective mechanical ventilation, taking an open lung approach in RDS may achieve desired results [2, 7]. As we mentioned previously, infants with RDS after recovering from asphyxia were treated with conventional mechanic ventilation with the parameters of a PIP of 40 cmH_2O, a PEEP of 7–8 cmH_2O, and RR of 70 breaths/min when various treatment measures were ineffective (note: such high ventilation parameters were considered only in a very few special cases). (3) Because of the seriousness of this condition, longer conventional mechanical ventilation treatment is needed, usually lasting over 10 days. Removing the ventilator within 7 days is very rare. Early removal of the ventilator will result in repeated need for the ventilator or recurrent disease and may even endanger the patient's life. (4) In terms of whether to use constant frequency ventilation or high-frequency ventilation, it depends on the conditions and personal experience. There is no fixed pattern for choosing which method to use; in particular, high-frequency ventilation cannot be regarded as an alternative mode of constant-frequency ventilation. Wunsch et al. conducted evidence-based medicine analysis of the relevant literature by searching in well-known databases, such as the Cochrane Library (2002, fourth edition), MEDLINE (1966–2002.10), EMBASE (1980–2002.11), World Wide Web, and Web of Science (1988–2002), at different times. The results showed that the effects of ALI and ARDS on the mortality and long-term morbidity were similar. We often encounter such a situation in clinic. The original effective ventilation in infants cannot maintain oxygenation without significant deterioration. Then, changing to high-frequency ventilation and oxygenation can result in short-term improvement, but this improvement very rapidly fails to be maintained. Then, if the constant frequency parameters are used (the same with parameters that were previously used), there may be short-term improvement in oxygenation status. This indicates that in treating extremely ill and hard-to-cure patients, constant frequency and high frequency can be used interchangeably. We have cured many such critically ill patients with this method, but the specific mechanism needs further study.
2. Exogenous pulmonary surfactant (EPS): Supplementing EPS is an important measure for successful rescue of full-term infants with RDS. EPS can significantly improve gas exchange, shorten the time of mechanical ventilation and prolong the survival time of patients with RDS, and reduce the mortality

of infants to some extent. However, in using EPS, one does not need to be particular about dosing; a small dose can achieve good results. We once encountered a critically ill patient. Under conditions of adequate ventilation parameters, NO inhalation, and high concentrations of oxygen inhalation, the patient's percutaneous oxygen saturation (SpO_2) could only be maintained at approximately 50–60%. After administering the full amount of EPS, SpO_2 could only be maintained at 60–70%. One EPS preparation at a time can raise SpO_2 to 60–70% in the short term. Thus, every time we gave the patient one EPS preparation, we repeated the administration every 6–8 h, and the patient's condition gradually improved, the SpO_2 rose gradually, and the patient finally recover and was discharged from hospital. For many reasons, many infants need repeated dosing of this medication: (1) The disease itself was too severe. (2) The start of treatment was too late. (3) The first treatment was seriously underdosed. (4) The pulmonary surfactant was inactivated. Inactivated pulmonary surfactant is an important reason for treatment failure or the need for repeated administration: (a) in the course of RDS treatment, especially in the late stage, the lung injury caused by various reasons can lead to the inactivation of PS; (b) the various components (plasma proteins, fibrinogen, etc.), inflammatory products (such as cytokines), and meconium particles in the plasma exudate after lung epithelial damage are the important causes of inactivation of PS; (c) the abovementioned factors can cause the decomposition of phospholipids, destroy the single molecular layer formed by PS on the alveolar surface, cause protein dissolution, destroy the synergistic effect of phospholipids and proteins, and eventually lead to PS inactivation.

3. Effective broad-spectrum antibiotics: Severe intrauterine infection is the first cause of RDS in full-term infants. Therefore, for infants with an onset of dyspnea shortly after birth, especially those with premature rupture of the fetal membranes, amniotic fluid III zero pollution, and mothers with a history of perinatal infection history, we first consider the disease secondary RDS caused by severe infection. While giving mechanical ventilation therapy, we also give broad-spectrum antibiotics to treat the infection and conduct dynamic monitoring of routine bloodwork, ESR, CRP, and routine blood cultures to guide antibiotic selection. However, although the infection is the first reason for RDS, laboratory evidence of infection within 24 h after birth is often inadequate, and routine bloodwork (white blood cell count, neutrophil percentage, and platelet count) and ESR and CRP anomalies are not significant but may become seriously and rapidly abnormal after 2–3 days.
4. Active treatment for persistent fetal circulation: Simple pulmonary hypertension (no right-to-left shunt) does not cause death, but if progression to a PFC occurs (presence of right-to-left shunt), the mortality will increase. For mild to moderate pulmonary hypertension in which there is no right-to-left shunt milrinone (first choice for patients with combined congenital heart disease) or magnesium sulfate (first choice for patients without congenital heart disease) can be given, an intravenous drip can provide a better therapeutic effect. For the treatment of the PFC, NO inhalation therapy is required. When NO is given, the concentration of oxygen inhalation can be reduced. Gitto et al. have proved that NO administered at a concentration <45% in NO inhalation is associated with reduced oxidative stress and inflammatory reaction. In cases in which no NO therapeutic equipment is available or in cases of poor responders to NO, give or combine the use of sildenafil. It should be emphasized that all patients should be evaluated with routine echocardiography in the meantime because in addition to complex congenital heart disease, changes in the pulmonary arterial pressure and the presence of PFC can be determined.
5. Active prevention and treatment of multiple organ failure: Patients tend to first developed PFC following RDS and ultimately develop multisystem organ failure and death. In the four cases of death with multiple organ failure, three cases had persistent fetal circulation. These four cases suffered from renal failure,

severe myocardial damage, and severe acidosis. Therefore, prevention and control of multiple organ failure is helpful to improve the patients' prognosis.

6. Nutrition and protection of the myocardium: (1) Due to infection, asphyxia and hypoxia, acidosis, hyperkalemia, and other factors, severe myocardial damage often occurs in full-term infants with RDS. (2) Myocardial damage is also an important cause of death in full-term infants with RDS. The four cases of death all presented with severe myocardial damage, including myocardial infarction and ventricular flutter or fibrillation. Therefore, protection of the myocardium and prevention of the occurrence of serious myocardial damage is an important aspect of treatment of full-term infants with RDS. Once the diagnosis is clear, myocardial nutritional medicine should be administered. Some commonly used medicines are 1,6-fructose diphosphate, large doses of vitamin C, etc.
7. Others: Correcting acidosis, disseminated intravascular coagulation, and low potassium are important factors to ensure the success of the treatment.
8. ECMO: This treatment will cure most patients, and patients who require ECMO therapy are very few. The development of ECMO in foreign countries has decreased, which is a sign of the progress of treatment technology. Invalid treatments are often performed in the following cases: a lack of knowledge of RDS in full-term infants; untimely ventilator treatment; unsuitable ventilator parameters; satisfactory oxygen synthesis in cases in which a head cover, CPAP, or lower mechanical ventilation parameters are used; premature ventilator withdrawal; and hereditary SP deficiency. When necessary, it is better to grasp the best opportunity to use ECMO; otherwise the purpose of treatment may not be achieved. It is generally considered that ECMO treatment should be given to infants with or without PPHN when the inhaled oxygen concentration is 1.3 and the oxygenation index is OI. Those suffering from fatal irreversible congenital anomalies are not suitable for ECMO treatment. In patients who have developed multiple organ failure, they have missed the opportunity for ECMO, and it is often unhelpful to carry out ECMO in these cases.
9. Lung transplantation: When infants with genetic SP deficiency develop respiratory failure at birth, they need immediate oxygen supply and conventional mechanical ventilation and often require extracorporeal membrane oxygenation, while exogenous pulmonary surfactant replacement therapy is often ineffective; moreover, if these patients do not undergo lung transplantation, they will die within 1 year.

In short, the pathogenesis of RDS in full-term infants, clinical characteristics, diagnosis, and treatment were briefly introduced. Although in full-term infants with RDS the fatality rate is higher, timely and appropriate treatment can significantly improve the prognosis. The treatment of full-term infants with RDS has no fixed or static model. Specific problems need specific treatment. In particular, the significant differences in etiology and pathogenesis prevent us from managing preterm infants with RDS similar to full-term infants with RDS; otherwise, there may be serious consequences.

3.3 Ultrasonographic Diagnosis of Respiratory Distress Syndrome

The ultrasonographic diagnosis of RDS is accurate; reliable; highly sensitive, with sensitivity of 100%; and specific. The ultrasound image displayed below shows pulmonary consolidation and air bronchograms, alveolar interstitial syndrome, abnormal pleural lines, decreased or absent lung sliding, absent lung islands, pleural effusion, lung pulses, and diffuse "white lung." When the three signs of pulmonary consolidation, pleural abnormalities, and diffuse "white lung" are present or disappear with A-lines, the sensitivity and specificity of RDS are 100% [7–13].

Pulmonary consolidation and the bronchial inflation sign are the most important ultrasound features of RDS. The extent and range of the consolidation is related to the extent of the disease. Mild RDS can be confined to small area of the pleural space. The local features and air bronchograms are not obvious in mild RDS, while the characteristics of severe RDS are very variable with a wide range of expansion. Pathologic changes are not only limited to the pleural space but also involve the deep lung. Air bronchograms are more obvious and can be located in different lung fields or limited to one side of the chest. The consolidated region and the surrounding lung tissue have no clear boundaries, but the affected area is easy to distinguish. Bronchial inflation is often fine, dense, and patchy.

"Bilateral white lung" or severe AIS is one of the most common features of RDS in ultrasound imaging. An ultrasound that shows "white lung" or AIS indicates the presence of lung edema. The more severe the pulmonary edema is, the degree of "white lung" or interstitial lung syndrome will be worse. Another important finding on lung ultrasound is that there is a pleural effusion in infants with RDS. The traditional view is that the main pathological feature of RDS is pulmonary atelectasis caused by a pulmonary surfactant deficiency. A chest X-ray may only display a uniform ground-glass change or "white lung," and it is very difficult to identify pleural effusion or pulmonary edema. However, the findings on lung ultrasound examinations have changed this traditional concept, that is, RDS may not only be associated with pulmonary atelectasis but also with pulmonary edema of different degrees and even pleural effusion. Therefore, compared with chest X-rays, lung ultrasonography provides us with more clinical and medical information, which helps to further enhance our understanding of RDS and contribute to the treatment of RDS. In the clinic, we often identify the same or similar common etiologies, individual data, clinical symptoms, and chest X-ray findings in infants, but they have a different response to the same treatment. The fundamental reason for this different response may lie in a difference in lung pathology. With an X-ray examination alone, it is difficult to distinguish between pathologies. What must be noted is that bilateral white lung or severe pulmonary syndrome alone is not enough to diagnose RDS. We must find pulmonary consolidation in certain parts of the lungs to distinguish RDS and TTN.

The morphology of the normal lung pleural line is smooth, and the width is not more than 0.5 mm; otherwise, it may be abnormal. For example, a rough, fuzzy, or irregular pleural line and a pleural thickness >0.5 mm, with pleural consolidation, are abnormal findings. The rate of abnormal findings in RDS is high, but other diseases, such as pneumonia, pulmonary hemorrhage, and TTN, can lead to pleural abnormalities. Therefore, it is not a specific change associated with RDS, and it is necessary to combine this finding with other ultrasound changes for diagnosis. The identification of a pleural abnormality has a sensitivity of 100% and a specificity of 45% for the diagnosis of RDS.

The A-lines that are present in normal lung tissue fail to be identified on lung ultrasound in infants with RDS, namely, the A-lines disappear. Other diseases can also lead to the reduction in or lack of A-lines, so this only hints lung lesions rather than being a specific change associated with RDS. However, a lack of A-lines coexists with lung consolidation and pleural abnormalities; both the sensitivity and specificity for RDS diagnosis reach 100%.

The lack of lung sliding on real-time ultrasound is another imaging feature of RDS that is often found in some infants with grade IV RDS. It is not common to find a pulmonary pulse, which is associated with consolidation and the condition of the lung.

In addition, we have also found that the double lung point can be identified during the acute stages of some mild RDS cases and during the recovery stages of some severe RDS cases. This finding is very different from previous opinions.

In summary, the most important indicator of RDS visualized by ultrasound is lung consolidation, which can be seen in all RDS patients; thus, we believe that if there is no consolidation, there is no RDS. However, the extent and scope of the lung consolidation vary with the grade of RDS. Among grade II RDS cases, the consolidation may be limited to the subpleural area, being focal and small-scale, and air bronchograms may be invisible. In contrast, the area of consolidation is significantly expanded in severe RDS (grades III–IV by chest X-ray), with air bronchograms becoming more obvious.

We stated that all the pictures or ultrasound images included in the chapter were taken from the Army General Hospital of the Chinese PLA and Beijing Chaoyang District Maternal and Child Healthcare Hospital; the related studies were approved by both the committee of the Army General Hospital and Chaoyang District Maternal and Child Healthcare Hospital.

Traditionally, RDS is characterized by atelectasis, even if it is severe RDS, which appears only as a "white lung" on a chest radiograph. In such a "white lung," it is difficult to visualize pleural effusion, pulmonary edema, or other pathological changes. Therefore, ultrasound findings have altered our traditional concepts. First, RDS exists not only with atelectasis but also with pulmonary edema or pleural effusion. Second, the extent and pathologic characteristics in the bilateral lungs can be inconsistent. These findings suggest that a lung ultrasound can provide us with additional medical and clinical information (Figs. 3.1, 3.2, 3.3, 3.4, 3.5, 3.6, 3.7, 3.8, 3.9, 3.10, 3.11, 3.12, 3.13, and 3.14).

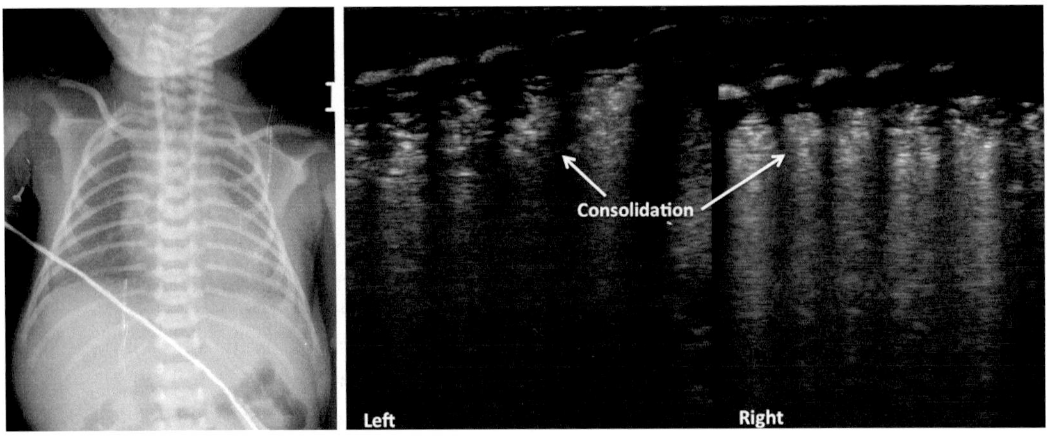

Fig. 3.1 Grade II RDS. Gestational age of 34^{+5} weeks, birth weight 2050 g. The patient was delivered by cesarean section, admitted for 4 h of dyspnea, and hospitalized 7 h after birth. A chest X-ray confirmed grade II RDS. A lung ultrasound showed bilateral consolidation with air bronchograms, with a lack of pleural lines and A-lines

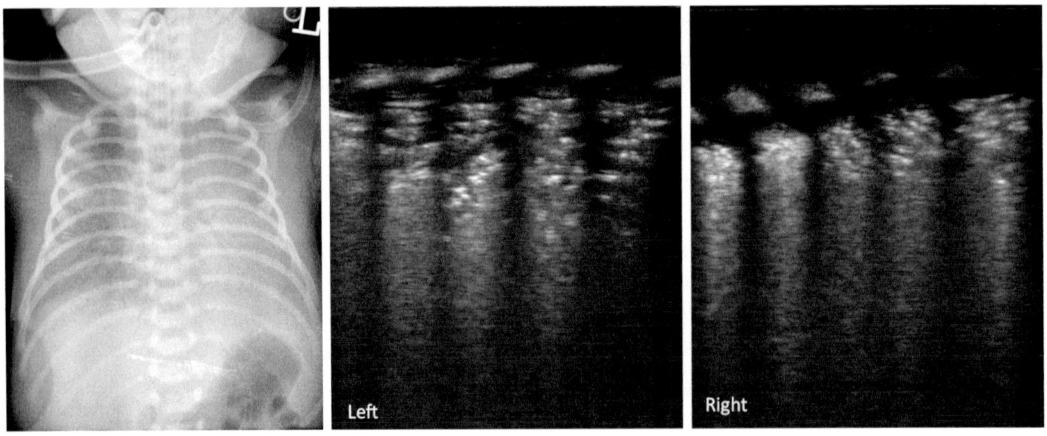

Fig. 3.2 Grade II-III RDS. G_2P_2, 37 W, 3250 g. The patient was delivered by natural labor, admitted for 4 h of progressive dyspnea, and hospitalized 4 h after birth. The clinical manifestations, arterial blood gas analysis, and chest X-ray examination confirmed a diagnosis of RDS. A chest X-ray showed that the lung penetration was significantly reduced, and the heart shadow was blurred, but the heart contour could still be distinguished. The symptoms were in accordance with the changes of grades II-III RDS. A lung ultrasound showed bilateral consolidation with air bronchograms, with a lack of pleural lines and A-lines

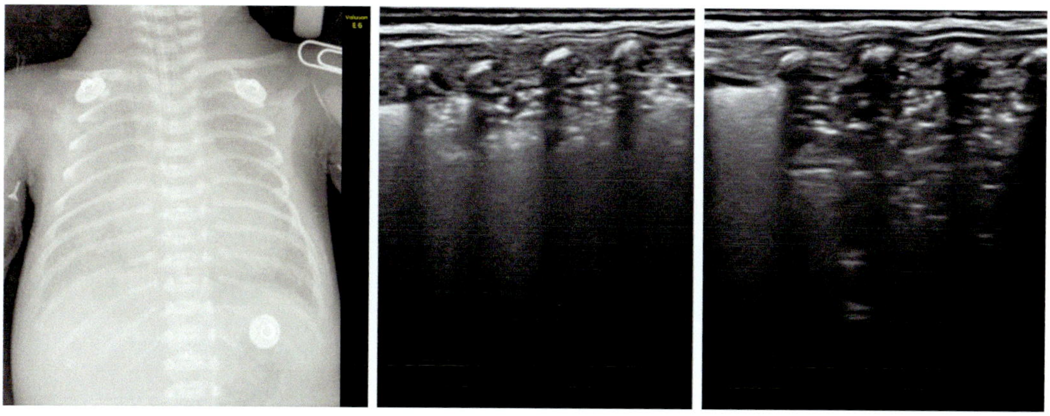

Fig. 3.3 Grade III RDS. G_1P_1, gestational age of 37^{+3} weeks, cesarean section delivery, birth weight 3100 g. The patient had dyspnea for 28 h and was hospitalized 28 h after birth. A chest radiograph showed grade IV RDS changes, and an ultrasound showed a large area of consolidation in the lung field with a significant bronchial aerate sign. There was a lack of pleural lines and A-lines

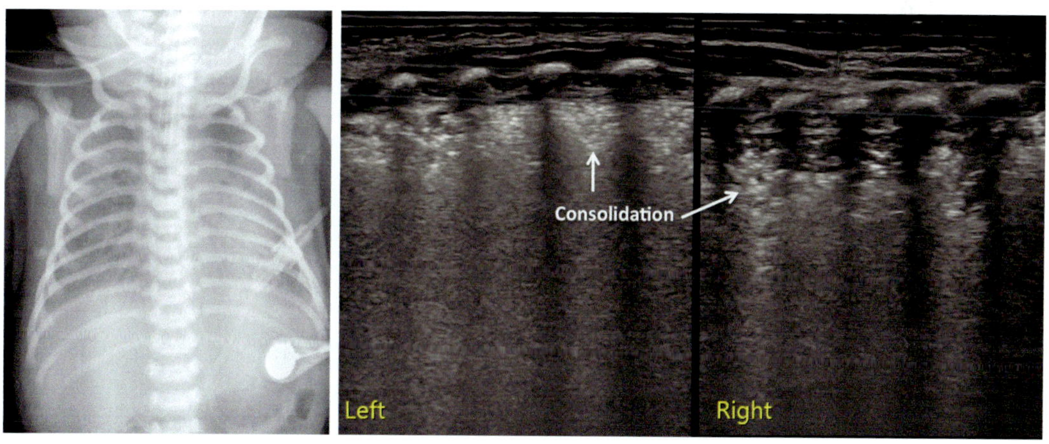

Fig. 3.4 Ultrasonographic findings in an RDS patient. The infant had a gestational age of 39^{+4} weeks and was delivered by cesarean section with a birth weight of 2970 g. The patient was admitted to the hospital because of dyspnea for 7 h after birth and diagnosed with RDS. An LUS showed a large area of lung consolidation with air bronchograms bilaterally and a lack of pleural lines and A-lines

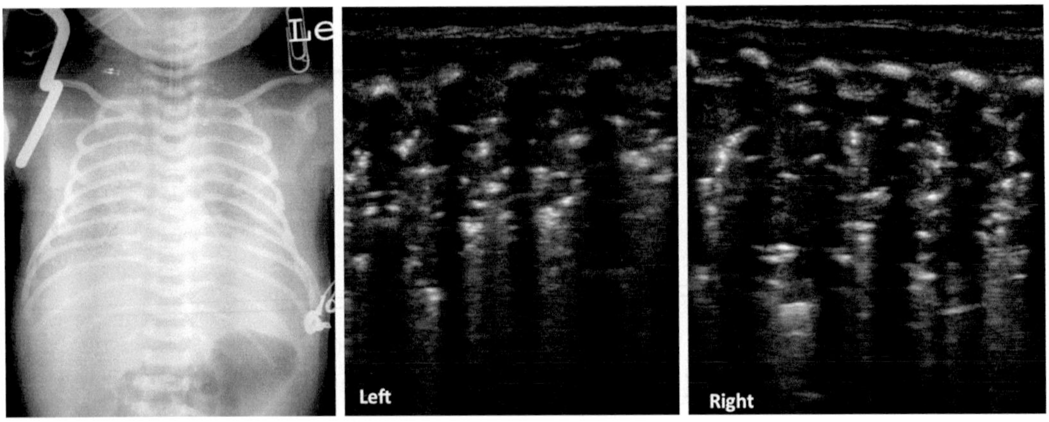

Fig. 3.5 Grade IV RDS. G_1P_1, gestational age of 40 weeks, birth weight 4440 g. The patient presented with severe asphyxia and was intubated. After the application of positive pressure ventilation and the administration of epinephrine and naloxone, the Apgar score was 2-3-8/1-5-10 min. The patient was admitted for progressive dyspnea for 10 h after recovering from asphyxia. A chest X-ray showed grade IV RDS changes. A lung ultrasound showed a large area of consolidation in the lung with an obvious bronchial inflation sign

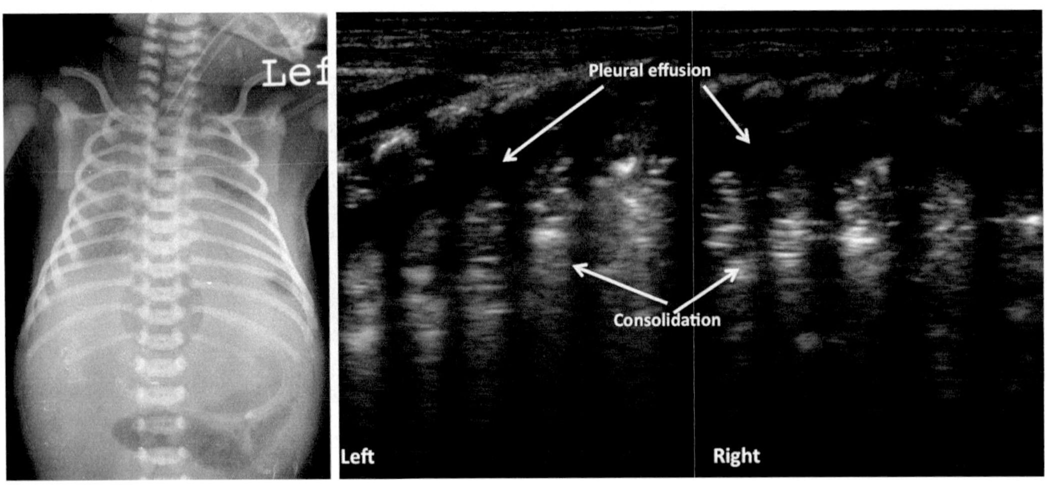

Fig. 3.6 Consolidation with bilateral pleural effusion in an RDS patient. Pleural effusion is a common ultrasonographic finding in RDS patients. It was never previously known that RDS could be associated with pleural effusion until ultrasound was used in the diagnosis of lung diseases. A chest X-ray showed grades II–III RDS, and a lung ultrasound showed significant bilateral lung consolidation with pleural effusion

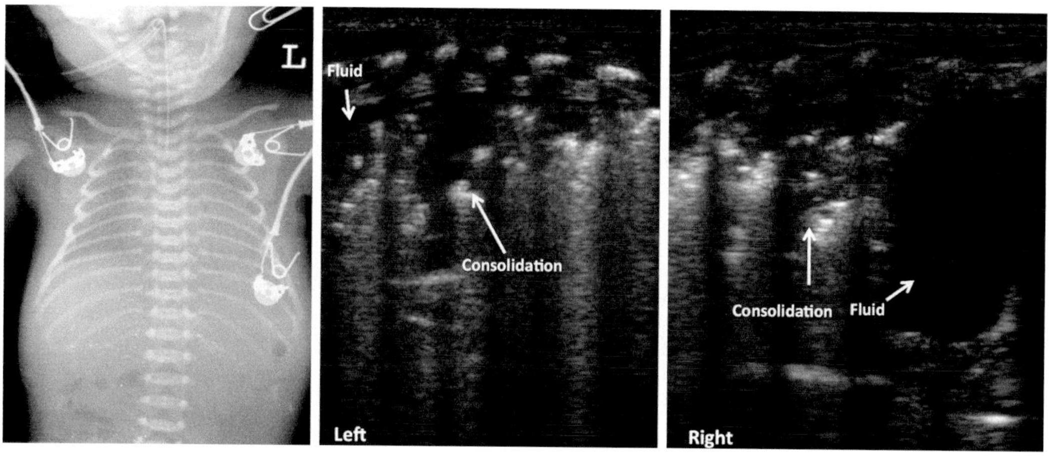

Fig. 3.7 Consolidation with bilateral pleural effusion in an RDS patient. The patient was clinically diagnosed with RDS according to the history, clinical manifestations, blood gas changes, and chest X-ray findings. An ultrasound showed significant consolidation in the upper field and pleural effusion in lower field of the right lung

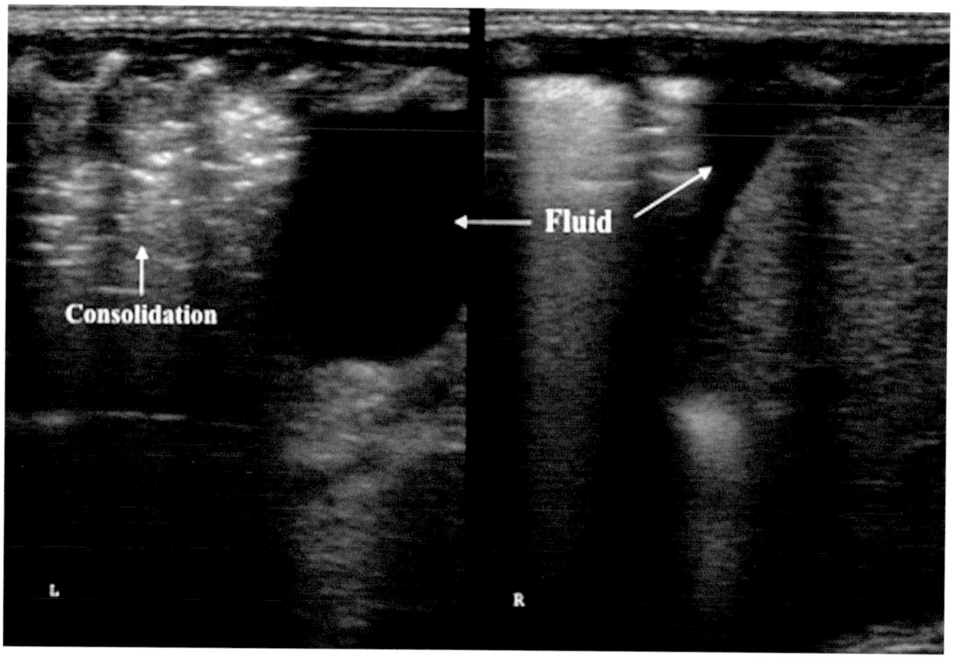

Fig. 3.8 Consolidation with bilateral pleural effusion. Gestational age 34^{+4} weeks, birth weight 1990 g. The patient was clinically diagnosed with RDS. A lung ultrasound showed bilateral pleural effusion (more significantly affecting the left lung), a large area of consolidation in the left upper lung field, and edema in the right upper lung field

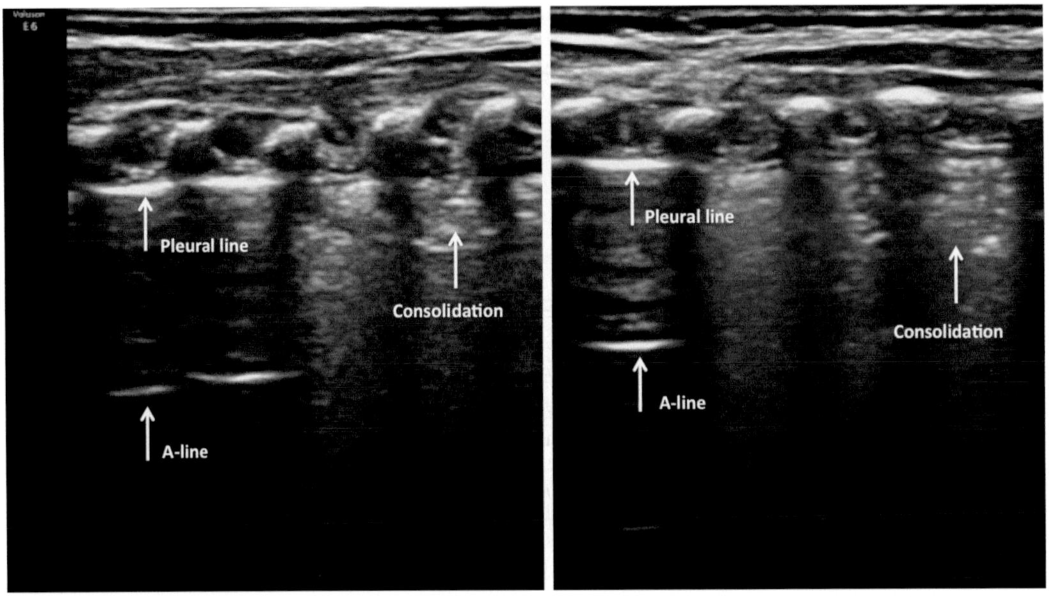

Fig. 3.9 Ultrasound findings in a mild RDS patient. Consolidation is the most important and major ultrasound manifestation of RDS. In mild RDS patients, however, the consolidation can be located in different areas of one lung field, while the other lung field remains normal

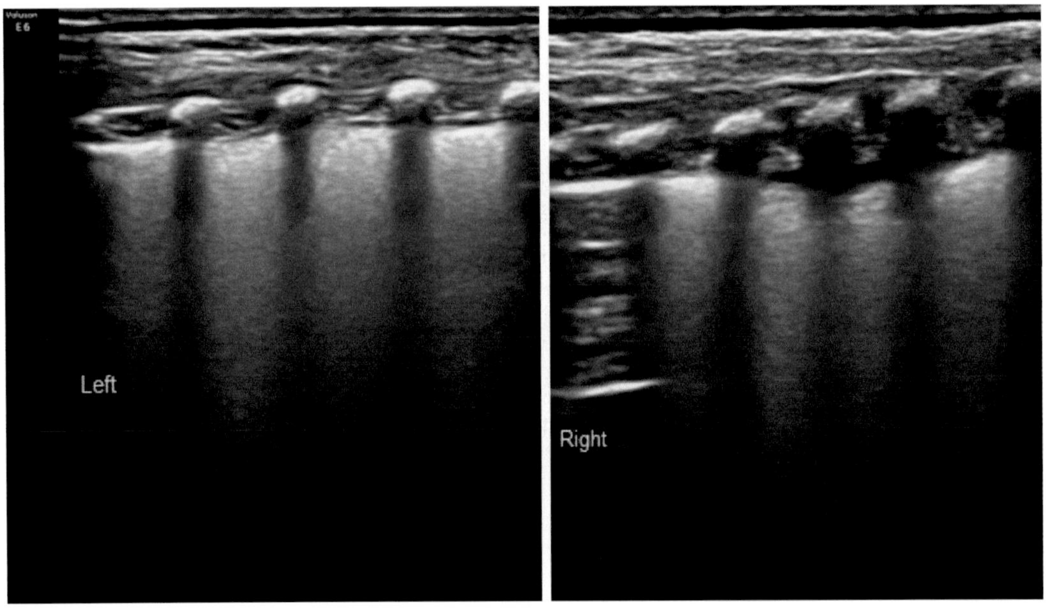

Fig. 3.10 Ultrasonographic findings in mild RDS. Consolidation can be inconspicuous, as in this patient, but it must exist in RDS patients; we believe that if there is no consolidation, there is no RDS. The picture shows mild bilateral consolidation and slight fluid in the right chest, with a lack of pleural lines and A-lines in the consolidated areas

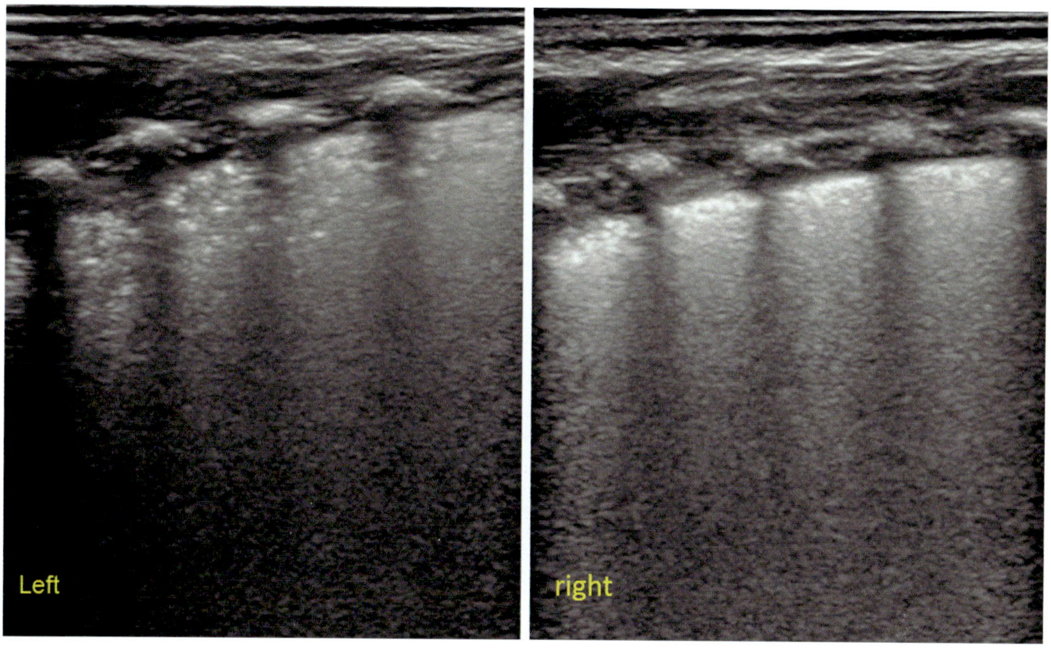

Fig. 3.11 Ultrasonographic manifestations of mild RDS. In mild RDS patients, the degree of consolidation can be insignificant. This is a grade II RDS patient according to chest X-ray and clinical manifestations, and the ultrasound image shows mild consolidation in the left lung and mild subpleural consolidation in the right lung

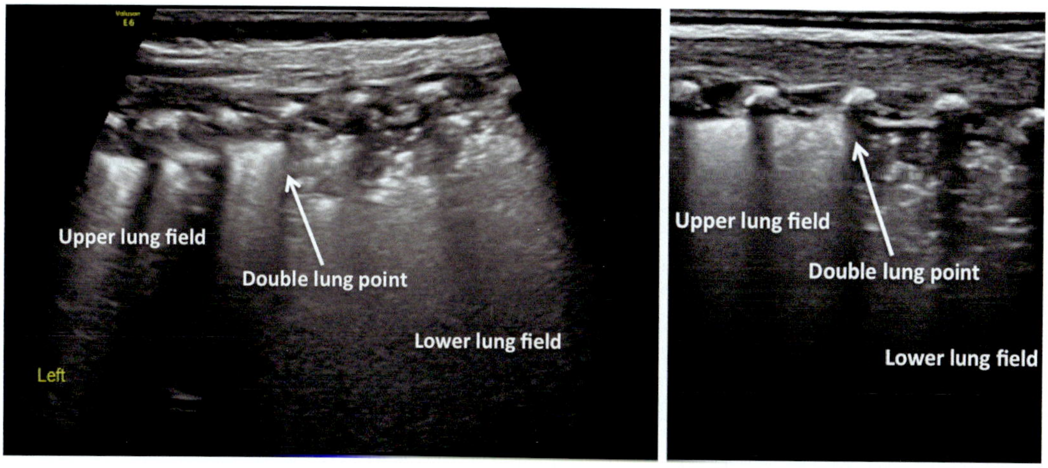

Fig. 3.12 Double lung point in RDS patients. It was believed that the double lung point (DLP) was the specific sign of wet lung, but we found that DLP could also be found in RDS and other lung diseases. This picture shows DLP in two different RDS patients. It can be seen that the upper lung field mainly manifested as AIS, while the lower lung field mainly manifested as consolidation with air bronchograms. The point between the upper and lower lung fields is the DLP

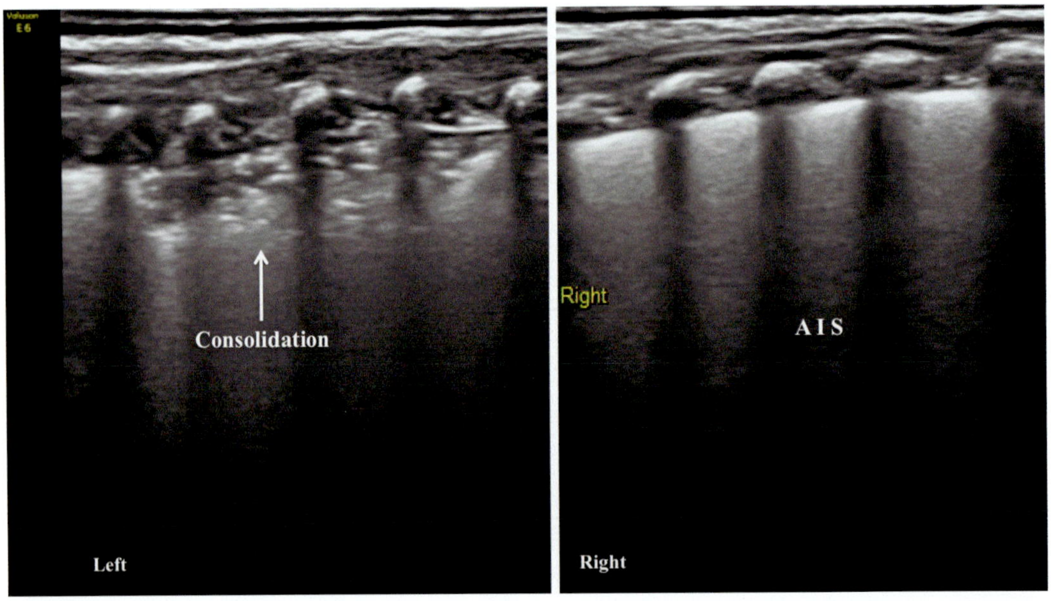

Fig. 3.13 Different ultrasonographic findings in the bilateral lungs. In RDS patients, the pathologic degree and the properties can be different in the bilateral lungs. The ultrasound image shows the double lung point and consolidation in different fields of the left lung in an RDS patient. This is grades II-III RDS patient according to chest X-ray manifestations, and the ultrasound image shows significant consolidation in the left lung and AIS in the right lung

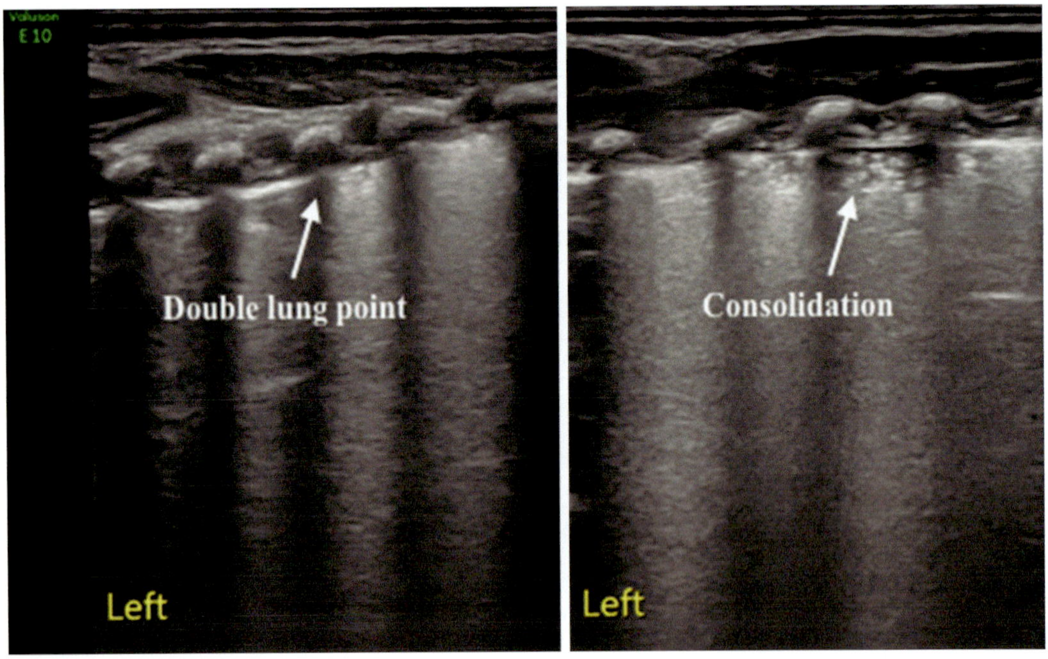

Fig. 3.14 Different ultrasonographic findings in the bilateral lungs. In RDS patients, the pathologic degree and the properties can be different in the bilateral lungs. The ultrasound image shows the double lung point and consolidation in different fields of the left lung in an RDS patient. This is a grade II RDS patient according to chest X-ray manifestations, and the ultrasound image shows the DLP in the left lung and mild consolidation in the right lung

References

1. Koivisto M, Marttila R, Kurkinen-Raty M, et al. Changing incidence and outcome of infants with respiratory distress syndrome in the 1990's: a population-based survey. Acta Paediatr. 2004;93(2):177–84.
2. Ayachi A, Rigourd V, Kieffer F, et al. Hyaline membrane disease in full-term neonates. Arch Pediatr. 2005;12(2):156–9.
3. Bouziri A, Ben Slima S, Hamdi A, et al. Acute respiratory distress syndrome in infants at term and near term about 23 cases. Tunis Med. 2007;85(10):874–9.
4. Berthelot-Ricou A, Lacroze V, Courbiere B, et al. Respiratory distress syndrome after elective caesarean section in near term infants: a five year cohort study. J Matern Fetal Neonatal Med. 2012;26:176. https://doi.org/10.3109/14767058.2012.733743.
5. Liu J, Shi Y, Dong JY, et al. Clinical characteristics, diagnosis and management of respiratory distress syndrome in full-term neonates. Chin Med J. 2010;123(19):640–2644.
6. Liu J, Yang N, Liu Y. High-risk factors of respiratory distress syndrome in term neonates: a retrospective case-control study. Balkan Med J. 2014;31(1):64–8.
7. Liu J, Chen XX, Li XW, et al. Lung ultrasonography to diagnose transient tachypnea of the newborn. Chest. 2016;149(5):1269–75.
8. Bober K, Swietliński J. Diagnostic utility of ultrasonography for respiratory distress syndrome in neonates. Med Sci Monit. 2006;12(10):CR440–6.
9. Cattarossi L, Copetti R, Macagno F, et al. Lung ultrasound in respiratory distress syndrome: a useful tool for early diagnosis. Neonatology. 2008;94(1):52–9.
10. Lovrenski J. Lung ultrasonography of pulmonary complications in preterm infants with respiratory distress syndrome. Ups J Med Sci. 2012;117(1):10–7.
11. Liu J, Cao HY, Wang HW, et al. The role of lung ultrasound in diagnosis of respiratory distress syndrome in newborn infants. Iran J Pediatr. 2014;24(2):147–54.
12. Liu J, Wang Y, Fu W, et al. The diagnosis of neonatal transient tachypnea and its differentiation from respiratory distress syndrome using lung ultrasound. Medicine. 2014;93(27):e197.
13. Cattarossi L, Copetti R. The "double lung point": an ultrasound sign diagnostic of transient tachypnea of the newborn. Neonatology. 2007;91(3):203–9.

Transient Tachypnea of the Newborn

4

Jing Liu, Hai-Ying Cao, and Erich Sorantin

4.1 Transient Tachypnea of the Newborn

Transient tachypnea of the newborn (TTN), also known as wet lung of the newborn, is one of the most common respiratory diseases of the newborn. TTN is self-limited with a good prognosis and low fatality and can be naturally recovered without any special intervention within 24–72 h in most cases. However, TTN can cause severe dyspnea, hypoxemia, pneumothorax, etc. TTN is the most common reason for dyspnea of the newborn. The incidence is 4–5.7% in full-term newborns and 10% in preterm infants, accounting for approximately 33–50% of dyspnea of the newborn [1, 2]. TTN is also often misdiagnosed as other diseases, especially among premature infants, as RDS, which can lead to overtreatment. According to *Neonatal Respiratory Disorders*, 77% of infants who were clinically diagnosed as RDS were actually TTN cases [1]. Therefore, it is necessary to pay more attention to this disease.

4.1.1 Morbidity and High-Risk Factors

The exact incidence of TTN is unclear. It is estimated that 0.33–0.5% of newborns suffer from wet lung when they are born. According to some epidemiological studies, the incidence of TTN of full-term newborns and premature infants is 4–5.7% and 10%, respectively. The main high-risk factors include cesarean section, large birth weight, maternal diabetes, maternal asthma, twins, male babies, apneic hypoxia, aspiration of amniotic fluid, overtransfusion after birth, delayed umbilical cord ligation, patent ductus arteriosus (left-to-right shunt and increased pulmonary blood flow increases hydrostatic pressure within blood capillaries of pulmonary vessels, which affects lung fluid clearance), hypoproteinemia, premature birth (a low level of noradrenaline, poor sensibility of β-adrenoceptor, and deficiency of pulmonary surfactant in the premature blood may damage the alveolar walls, influencing lung fluid clearance; low plasma protein leads to malabsorption of lung fluid; in addition, factors such as small premature thoraxes, weak respiratory muscles, poor pulmonary compliance, and small gas exchange areas delay lung fluid absorption), etc. [1–4].

Electronic Supplementary Material The online version of this chapter (https://doi.org/10.1007/978-94-024-1549-0_4) contains supplementary material, which is available to authorized users.

J. Liu (✉)
Department of Neonatology and NICU,
Beijing Chaoyang District Maternal and Child Health Care Hospital, Beijing, China

H.-Y. Cao
Department of Ultrasound, GE Healthcare, Beijing, China

E. Sorantin
Division of Pediatric Radiology, Department of Radiology, Medical University Graz, Graz, Austria

J. Liu et al. (eds.), *Neonatal Lung Ultrasonography*, https://doi.org/10.1007/978-94-024-1549-0_4

4.1.2 Pathogenesis

Fetal lungs are filled with fluid secreted by alveolar epithelial cells in utero. Active Cl^- of alveolar epithelial cells enters into the alveolar space to promote lung fluid secretion (low absorption of Na^+) and adjust the growth and development of lungs in reverse. The alveolar liquid enters into the amniotic fluid via tracheal bronchi by fetal respiratory movements. During the last trimester of pregnancy and a short time before delivery, the secretion fluid of fetal lungs is transformed into absorption fluid. At this time, due to the increase in Na^+ channels of alveolar epithelial cells, nonpreference of activities of ion channels is transformed into high selectivity of Na^+ so that Na^+ absorption increases significantly. With the reabsorption of Na^+, large amounts of lung fluid are absorbed. After birth, reabsorption of Na^+ increases significantly (accompanied with Cl^- reabsorption), which rapidly changes the state of fetal lungs from plentiful fluid secretion to little lung fluid. Generally, it takes approximately 6 h to clear the fluid in the lungs completely after birth. If the clearance is delayed, TTN may occur [1–4].

It is believed that there are two main mechanisms of lung fluid clearance, namely, Na^+ pumps and mechanical force. The enhancement of Na^+ pump activity is the main mechanism. Under the effect of sodium-potassium ATPase, Na^+ passes through epithelial Na^+ channels (ENaCs) located in type I and II epithelial cells and cyclic nucleotide-gated channels (CNGCs) on type I epithelial cells from the top surface and enters into the intercellular space from the surface of the basal membrane and cytomembrane. During these events, H_2O is reabsorbed, and ions also form a significant osmotic gradient by transferring aquaporins (AQP) from alveolar epithelial cells or diffusion to promote the absorption of the lung field. AQP has many subtypes, and its role in fetal absorption of the lung field is not the same as its role in the adult lung. Compared with adults, the expression of AQP1 and AQP5 is higher at birth. Antepartum cortical hormones can increase the expression of AQP1 and AQP4 (with no influence on AQP5). A delivery enhances the expression of AQP4, and acidosis during the perinatal period restrains the expression of AQP3 [3].

At birth, the main behaviors of alveolar epithelial cells change from Cl^- secretion to Na^+ reabsorption with ENaC opening, constituting three subunits, α, β, and γ. Though the exact mechanism of lung field clearance at birth is not yet clear, activity decrease or immaturity of this process may lead to TTN during an impending delivery or initiation of a delivery. The Na^+ transfer within 1–4 h after birth is closely related to lung compliance within 21–48 h after birth. At birth, reabsorption of Na^+ increases the birth weight of newborns. The expression levels of ENaC α, β, and γ of premature respiratory tracts are lower than those of the respiratory tracts of full-term infants [3].

It is difficult to explain the significance of genetic predisposition of familial TTN. In a rat model, knockout of genes coding the α-subunit (genes coding the β- and γ-subunits were not affected) may damage the clearance function of lung fluid and lead to death due to severe dyspnea. ENaC gene mutation (in which a gene mutation of the α-subunit is the most common) of pseudohypoaldosteronism patients may cause pulmonary dysfunction of ENaC. Though the α-subunit coded by a gene polymorphism of the 12th and 13th exons is related to the susceptibility of TTN, the effects of genovariation of α-subunits on the susceptibility of TTN are unknown [3].

The regulation of Na^+ channels of pulmonary epithelial cells is not yet clear, but key factors may be oxygen, cortical hormones, and catecholamine. Low oxygen can restrain the activity of sodium-potassium ATPase to inhibit Na^+ transfer by ENaC. Glucocorticoids can increase Na^+ reabsorption of pulmonary epithelial cells by the following mechanisms: (1) stimulating the transcription of ENaC subunits to decrease the damage to ENaC, which increases the number of effective ENaC and enhances the activity of the original ENaC, and (2) promoting the reactivity of β-epinephrine and thyroxine. With a lack of oxygen and glucocorticoids, alveolar cells may primarily express nonselective ENaC comprised of α-subunits instead of transferring large amounts of Na^+. Consequently, not enough lung fluid is cleared at birth. Dexamethasone may prevent reabsorption of lung fluid caused by anoxia and stimulate the expression of transfer carriers of Na^+ (even under an anoxic condition) [3].

The most effective strategy to promote fetal lung absorption is to use exogenous cortical hormones. Thirty-seven- to thirty-eight-week-old fetuses who experience an elective cesarean section receive a single course of cortical hormones 48 h before the procedure with the aim of significantly decreasing the incidence of respiratory diseases.

During a delivery, 25–35% of lung fluid can be lost through squeezing the thorax through the birth canal. Though the birth canal squeeze is considered the main pressure for lung fluid clearance, a change of fetus position due to constant uterine contraction during a delivery may also press the thorax. Therefore, there is a large amount of lung fluid of a puerpera in an elective cesarean section before the initiation of the delivery. The incidence of respiratory diseases of infants who experienced an elective cesarean section before 39 weeks increases by 4.1, 3.3, and 2.1 times. As a result, it is suggested that a puerpera who needs a cesarean section should have the procedure after 39 weeks of pregnancy.

During the last trimester of pregnancy, epinephrine is released largely to stimulate pulmonary epithelial cells to inhibit lung fluid secretion so lung fluid absorption can begin. A delivery (including cesarean sections) promotes lung fluid absorption in the fetus. If an infant is born after the initiation of a delivery, the incidence of TTN is low. However, recent research showed that cesarean section cannot prevent TTN after the initiation of a delivery, so the mechanism of a vagina during a delivery and even the rupture of fetal membranes may be necessary for TTN prevention.

More than 90% of β-adrenoceptors are located in pulmonary alveoli. Though both β_1- and β_2-adrenoceptors exist on alveolar walls, β_2-adrenoceptors are dominant (70%). β_2-adrenoceptors upregulate the activity of ENaC to enhance Na^+ transfer of pulmonary alveoli. Both animal experiments and clinical adult research have shown that inhalation or injection of β-adrenergic preparations can accelerate the clearance of lung fluid, suggesting the possibility of treating pneumonedema and acute lung injury with β-adrenergic preparations [1–3].

Changes in gene expression and performance of β-adrenoceptors caused by single nucleotide polymorphisms are involved in the pathogenesis of multiple lung diseases, including TTN and asthma. The β-adrenergic genetic predisposition and low reactivity can cause TTN and asthma in adults. Therefore, it is believed that TTN may be an initial symptom of asthma.

4.1.3 Clinical Manifestation

Infants mainly show dyspnea. At birth, most child patients were normal or had a history of asphyxia and had dyspnea a few hours (2–5 h) later. In some cases, dyspnea is not obvious, and their main manifestations are tachypnea, cyanosis, etc. without obvious hypoxia, while in severe cases, they showed severe respiratory distress, obvious tachypnea, cyanosis, splittle, and poor response but with a normal body temperature. There may be decreased breath sounds or coarse rales during lung auscultation.

Arterial blood gas analysis of most cases was normal, while hypercapnia, hypoxemia, and metabolic acidosis may occur among particularly severe patients.

TTN is self-limited with a good prognosis. In some cases, it can be recovered within 5–6 h or 1 day, while in severe cases, it takes 4–5 days to recover.

4.1.4 Manifestation of Chest X-Rays

1. Alveoli effusion signs: density, sizes, shapes, and distribution of lesions change with different contents of alveoli effusion. Its manifestations are as follows: (1) patchy shadows of different sizes, (2) small nodular shadows with diameters of 2–4 mm, and (3) veil-like or

ground-glass-like cloudy shadows and "white lung" changes in severe cases. These changes can occur singly or simultaneously. A pulmonary lobule was taken as a unit of localized lesions (in basal segments of lower lobes mostly due to newborn clinostatism and weight of fluid) or generalized, which is mainly distributed in the inner middle areas of both lung fields and lower lung fields with uniform distribution and more serious on the right side. Patients with severe clinical dyspnea and "white lung" change in X-rays are often misdiagnosed as RDS.
2. Interstitial effusion signs: (1) X-rays show netlike and stripe-like shadows, indicating that fluid is accumulated in the alveolar septum, interlobular septum, and peripheries of bronchi and blood vessels. (2) Interlobar pleural effusion: interlobar fractures manifest as band-like or fusiform broadening shadows; a few pleural effusions manifest as strip-like shadows in the inner edge of the chest wall with a lack of costophrenic angles.
3. Other manifestations are (1) increased, thickened, and blurred lung markings, radiating from the hilum of the lung and extending outward, due to expanded lymphatic vessels and pulmonary veins around the blood vessels and (2) emphysema—increased transparency of the lung field due to compensatory enlargement of inflatable alveoli.

Alveoli effusion and interlobar pleural effusion are the most common and earliest signs of TTN on X-rays, and they are characterized by graininess, small patchy shadows, patchy shadows of extensive fusion, and net or filiform dense shadows. Pulmonary congestion and emphysema are also common. Thickening of the pleura and pleural effusion accounted for 26.2% of cases, and enlargement of heart shadows and broadening of mediastina accounted for 35.7%. Lung X-rays of TTN showed that 71% absorption was reached within 24 h and 97.8% absorption was completed within 72 h. The minority of cases had delayed absorption for 4 days. Absorption of pulmonary lesions started from the periphery, and they were absorbed from the upper lung field to the lower lung field gradually. With adjustment and recovery of physiological functions of the lungs, the congestion of pulmonary vessels tends to change over time. Therefore, pulmonary hemangiectasis due to congestion tends to occur during absorption of lung alveolar fluid and become more significant within 24–36 h after birth. With absorption of alveolar fluid, the alveolar volume declines gradually, and pulmonary interstitial effusion becomes more significant with short-term (8–10 h) netlike shadows. Of note, TTN may coexist with other diseases, so X-ray evidence of other relevant diseases should be considered.

4.1.5 Differential Diagnosis

TTN needs to be distinguished from many diseases, RDS and intrauterine infection pneumonia, as shown in the following table (Table 4.1).

4.1.6 Treatment

The main treatments are increased care and symptomatic treatment. When tachypnea and cyanosis are obvious, patients are given oxygen therapy and undergo arterial blood gas analysis. Respirators should be provided for assisted respiration if necessary. Patients with metabolic acidosis can be treated by intravenous drip of sodium bicarbonate, dysphoria by phenobarbital sodium, and excessive moist rales by furosemide. Various complications should be considered.

4.2 Ultrasound Diagnosis of Transient Tachypnea of the Newborn

Using ultrasound to diagnose TTN is simple, convenient, accurate, and reliable. Double lung points are the most specific ultrasonic characteristic of mild TTN. The main manifestations in severe patients are severe pulmonary interstitial syndrome and diffuse white lung (namely, pneumonedema). Previously, it was believed that double lung points had 100% sensitivity and specificity for the diagnosis of TTN [5, 6].

Table 4.1 Distinction of TTN, RDS, and intrauterine infection pneumonia

	TTN	*RDS*	Intrauterine infection pneumonia
Gestational age	Premature or full term	Occurs in both premature and full-term infants	Premature or full term
Medical history	Cesarean section, maternal asthma	Premature delivery, elective cesarean section, perinatal infections, premature rupture of fetal membranes	Perinatal infections, premature rupture of fetal membranes
Pulmonary surfactant	Deficiency among premature puerperas	Primary or secondary deficiency	A possibility of primary or secondary deficiency
Dyspnea	Mostly slight	Mostly severe	May be slight or severe
Blood gas analysis	Mostly normal or PaO_2-reduced	Reduction in PaO_2, increase in $PaCO_2$ and acidosis	Reduction in PaO_2 and acidosis
Changes in chest X-rays	Alveoli effusion and interstitial effusion, thickening of lung markings	Reduction in transparency of lung fields, air bronchogram, and "white lungs"	Coarse, punctate, and flake-like shadows, involvement of one lobe or lung segments
Hemogram and CRP	Normal	Related to infections or increased	Increased
Mechanical ventilation	The majority does not need mechanical ventilation	The majority needs mechanical ventilation and oxygen supply	Severe patients need mechanical ventilation
Course of disease	The majority are resolved within 72 h	The majority lasts more than 7 days	The majority lasts 10–14 days
Prognosis	Good	High mortality rate	Mostly good

However, with experience and an increased understanding of lung ultrasounds, we found that this was not always the case. Double lung points are related to water content of the upper and lower lung fields, and severe pneumonedema shows no sign of double lung points. Due to severe pneumonia edema at the early stage of the disease, many patients show pulmonary interstitial syndrome or diffuse white lung on their lung ultrasound images. However, with disease progression and the clearance of lung fluid, double lung points gradually disappear. This phenomenon also occurs in other lung diseases, such as RDS, pneumonia, and pneumorrhagia [7]. Other common manifestations include pleural effusion, abnormalities of the pleura line, disappearance of A-lines, etc. There is no lung consolidation when patients suffer from TTN. However, lung consolidation of various degrees occurs when patients suffer from diseases such as RDS and MAS. Therefore, if lung consolidation is found by ultrasound, TTN can be excluded [6, 7].

The main pathomechanism of TTN is the increase in water content within the lung tissue. The mechanisms of comet tail signs, B-lines, AIS, and "white lung," are the same and are related to the increase in water within the lung tissue. Low water content manifests as comet tail sign or B-lines. Intensive B-lines further form AIS, and severe AIS is "white lung." Thus, "white lung" and AIS are important changes in an ultrasonogram indicating pneumonedema and were seen in each TTN patient. However, "white lung" and AIS can also be observed in other lung diseases resulting in water increase within lung tissue, such as RDS and MAS. Therefore, "white lung" and AIS are necessary and nonspecific to TTN [7].

The abnormality of the pleura line is a common change in ultrasound images due to TTN. Abnormalities of the pleura line include thickening, blurring, disappearing pleura lines, etc., which are related to degrees of pneumonedema. Simultaneously, the disappearance of A-lines can be observed. According to the generation mechanism, A-lines are reverberation artifacts formed by echoes of pleura lines. Therefore, an abnormality of a pleura line must accompany the disappearance of A-lines. However, a change of A-lines is affected by the water content of the lung tissue. Therefore, when patients suffer from TTN, a disappearance or reduction of A-lines is more common than abnormalities of pleura lines. Likewise, abnormalities of pleura lines and the disappearance of A-lines can be observed in other lung diseases. Thus, they are not specific signs of TTN.

TTN often accompanies pleural effusion, which can be easily observed during ultrasound examination. Wet lung is one of the common causes of pleural effusion in newborns. Therefore, pleural effusion discovered by ultrasound has some reference value to further diagnose wet lung. For TTN, ultrasound features of different lung fields may be significantly different. Not only can ultrasound features of both sides of the lungs be different, but also those of one side can be inconsistent. Thus, ultrasound features, such as double lung points, are generated. This phenomenon indicates that water contents of the lung tissue (namely, degrees of pneumonedema) in different areas are inconsistent. Therefore, lung ultrasound examinations are conducive to further understanding lung diseases.

Though TTN is clinically common, it is difficult to distinguish it from other diseases correctly. TTN is often misdiagnosed as other lung diseases such as RDS. Especially in premature infants accompanied with (1) respiratory distress with expiration moan; (2) significantly abnormal blood gas; and (3) a chest X-ray showing a "white" or nearly "white" lung, TTN is often misdiagnosed as RDS. It is considered that 77% of infants who have been diagnosed with RDS actually suffer from TTN [1], which is a high misdiagnosis rate. However, ultrasound examination contributes to the differential diagnosis of TTN and RDS. Pulmonary consolidation and air bronchogram are not observed by ultrasound of TTN patients. According to literature reports, all RDS patients have pulmonary consolidation and air bronchogram [6–8]. Therefore, pulmonary consolidation and air bronchogram are important for the differential diagnosis of TTN and RDS. Similar problems often occur clinically. Patients, who are sick and hospitalized due to dyspnea and have especially fuzzy cardiac borders or "white lung" discovered by chest X-ray examination, are often diagnosed as RDS and accept the corresponding treatment. After we performed a lung ultrasound examination, we found that some infant patients had no "pulmonary consolidation or air bronchogram" and only showed severe pneumonedema or complicated pleural effusion and features of double points. Therefore, they are TTN instead of RDS [6–8].

Our findings are illustrated in Figs. 4.1, 4.2, 4.3, 4.4, 4.5, 4.6, 4.7, 4.8, 4.9, 4.10, and 4.11. We stated that all the pictures or ultrasound images

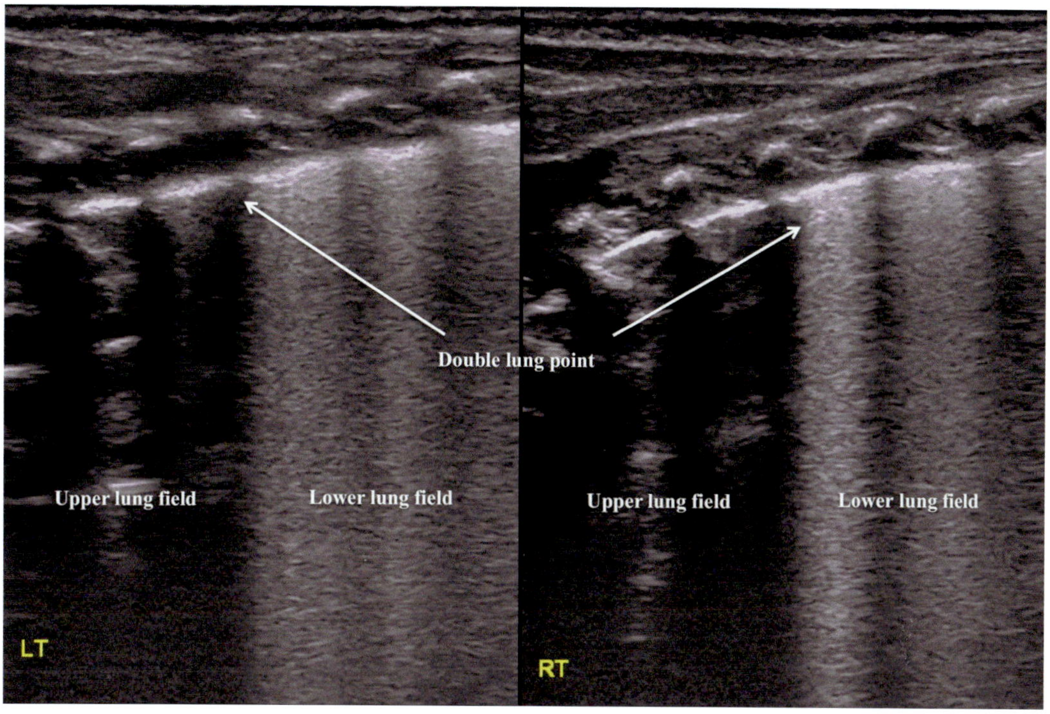

Fig. 4.1 Double lung point in TTN. G_1P_2, 40 weeks of gestation, vaginal delivery, a birth weight of 2870 g. The patient was admitted to the hospital due to tachypnea after birth for 2 h. Obvious double lung points in bilateral lungs were shown by lung ultrasound accompanied with thickened and blurred pleural lines and a lack of A-lines. The double lung point is often seen in mild TTN patients

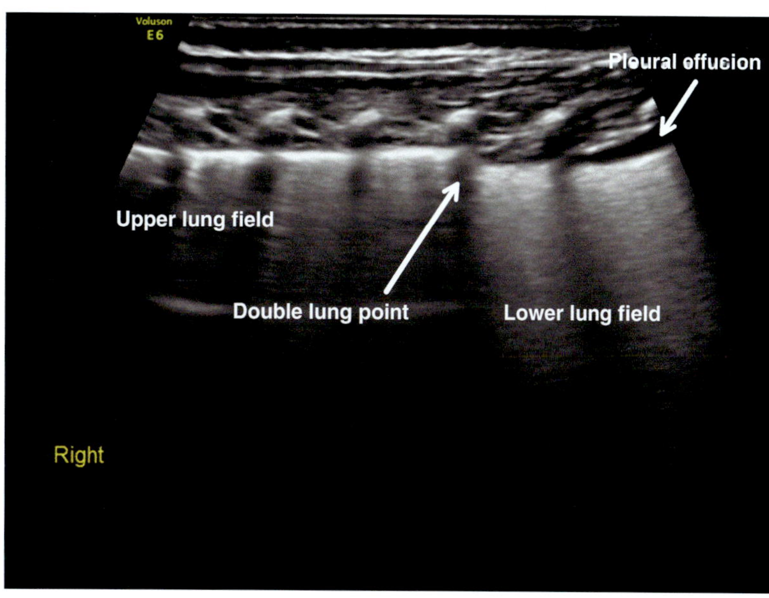

Fig. 4.2 Double lung point in TTN. During ultrasonography, the lung field echoes clearly differ from the upper to lower lung. This demarcation point is called the double lung point in a mild TTN patient. Less pleural effusion was observed in this patient's lower lung field

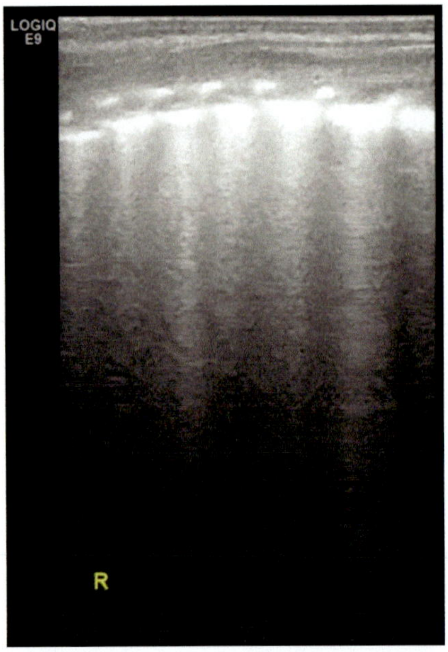

Fig. 4.3 AIS in TTN. Lung AIS was identified by the presence of more than two B-lines within each lung field. The pleural line was abnormal, and the A-line disappeared; however, the acoustic shadows of the ribs may be present. This is one of the common nonspecific manifestations of mild-to-moderate TTN

included in the chapter were taken from the Army General Hospital of the Chinese PLA and Beijing Chaoyang District Maternal and Child Healthcare Hospital; the related studies were approved by both the committee of the Army General Hospital and Chaoyang District Maternal and Child Healthcare Hospital.

TTN can also develop into RDS (or TTN can also lead to RDS). Thus, it is important to conduct follow-up examinations when a patient with respiratory distress is administered to a NICU (Fig. 4.12).

In conclusion, according to our studies and experience, severe TTN primarily manifests as white lung or a compact B-line, whereas mild TTN primarily manifests as AIS or a double lung point. These findings contradict past opinions that both the sensitivity and specificity of identifying a double lung point in diagnosing TTN are 100%; instead, our findings indicate that white lung/compact B-line had a sensitivity of 33.8% and a specificity of 91.3% for diagnosing TTN, whereas double lung point had a sensitivity of 45.6% and a specificity of 94.8% for diagnosing severe TTN [7].

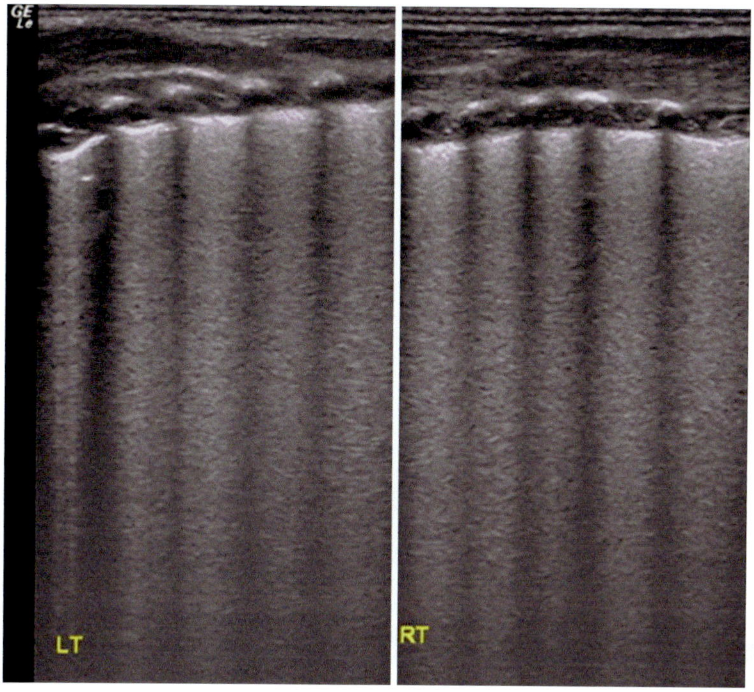

Fig. 4.4 AIS in TTN. The ultrasound showed that the pleural line was abnormal and the A-line disappeared. Therefore, this is AIS, which presented with lung edema. Lung edema is the main ultrasound manifestation of TTN and presents to varying degrees in different diseases

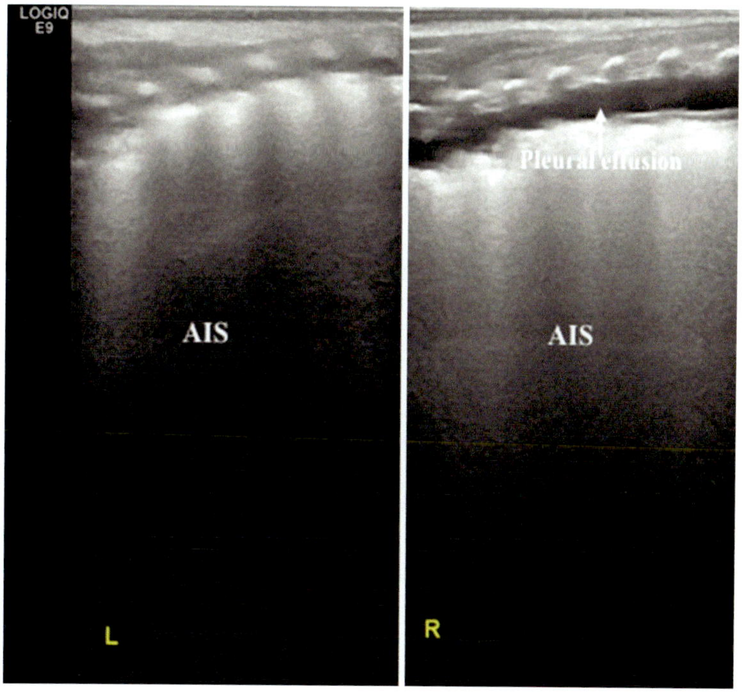

Fig. 4.5 AIS with pleural effusion in TTN. A more severe TTN patient. The left lung mainly presents as AIS, with a lack of A-lines and a blurred pleural line under ultrasound, while the right lung mainly presents as pleural effusion and disappeared A-lines and pleural line

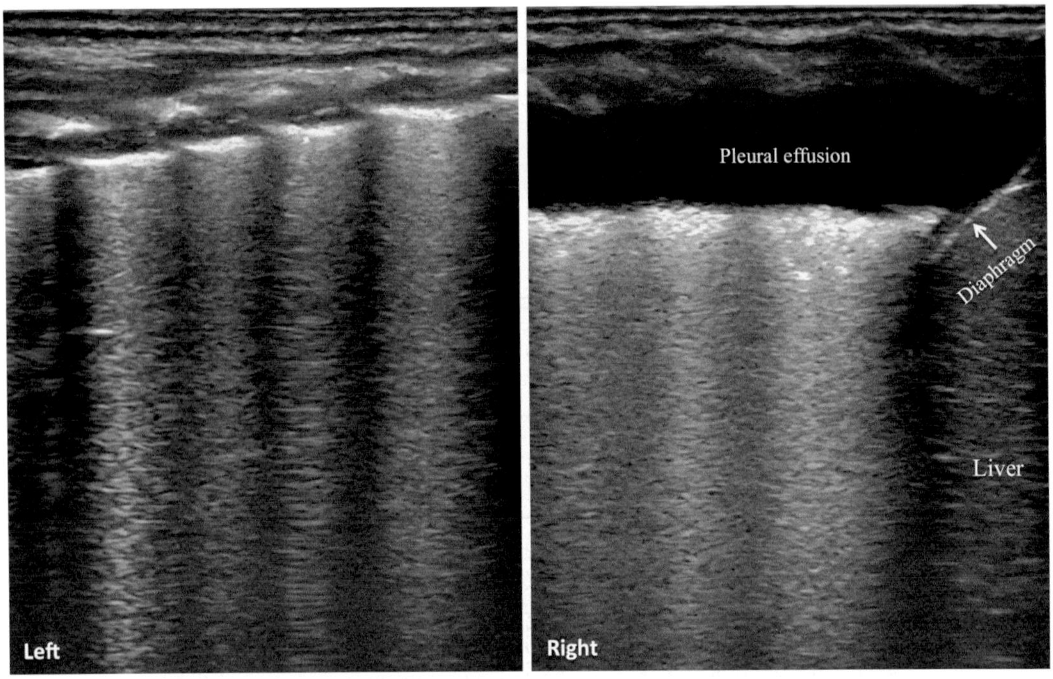

Fig. 4.6 AIS with pleural effusion in TTN. G_1P_1, 38 weeks, cesarean section with a birth weight of 3770 g. The patient was admitted to the hospital due to tachypnea for 4 h after birth. The blood gas analysis was almost normal. In addition to tachypnea, there were no obvious chest wall retractions or cyanosis. The lung ultrasound showed a disappearance of pleura lines and A-lines in both lungs and an "alveolar-interstitial syndrome-like" change in the bilateral lung field, indicating there were large amounts of fluid in this lung. There was an obvious dark area of fluid in the right lung, indicating pleural effusion. This finding showed that lesion degrees of wet lung in infant patients may be different in both lungs

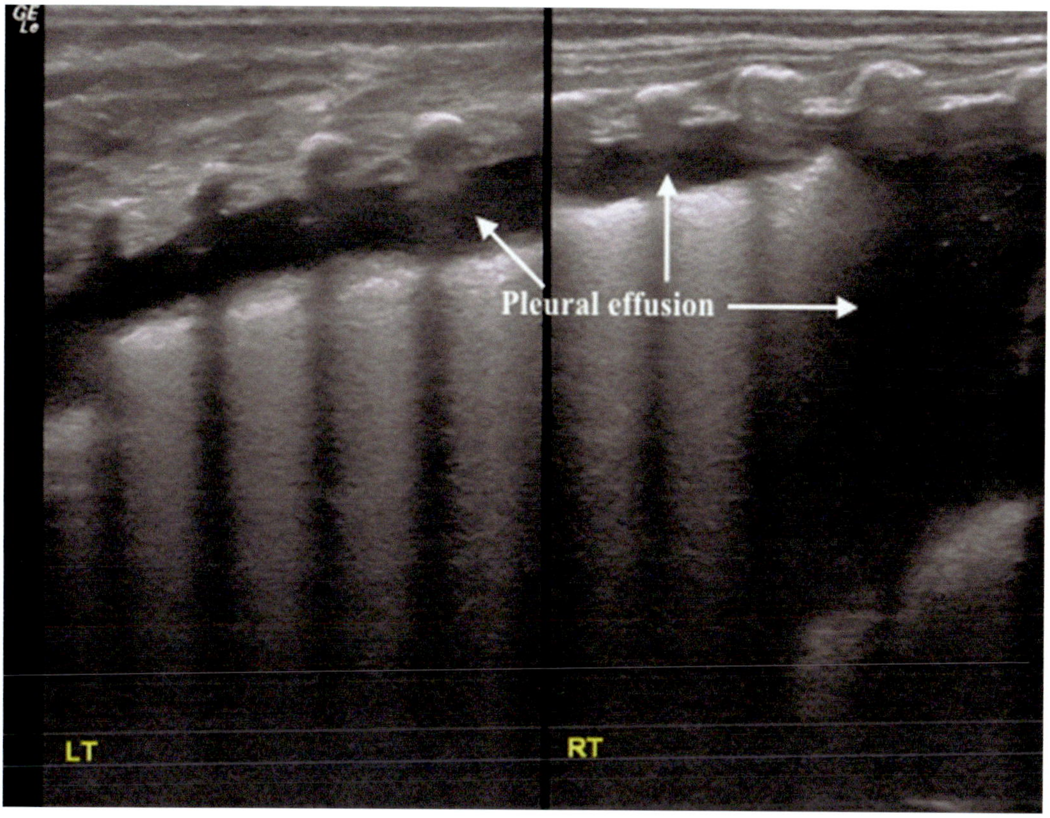

Fig. 4.7 Bilateral pleural effusion in TTN. Different degrees of pleural effusion are a common ultrasonic finding in TTN patients, which can be unilateral (Fig. 4.6) or bilateral (this case)

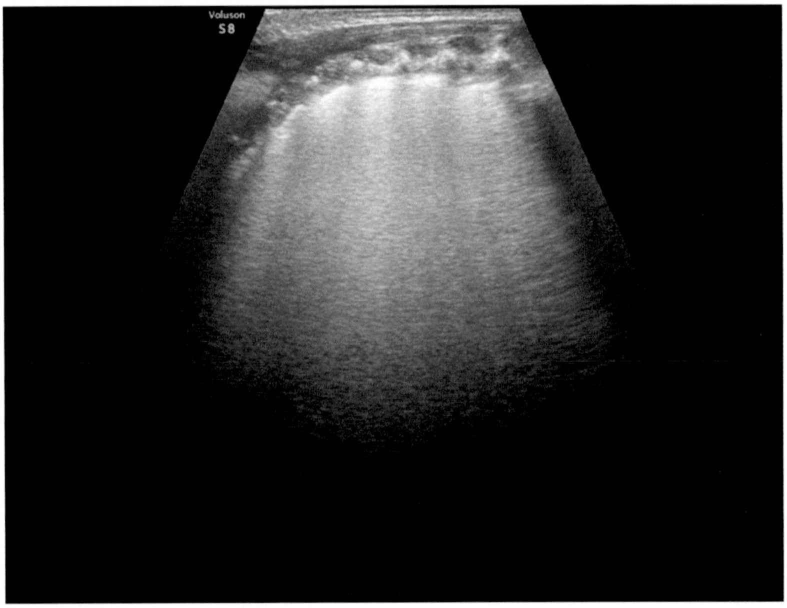

Fig. 4.8 Compact B-Line in a severe TTN patient. The probe is perpendicular to the ribs during the scan. The dense existing B-line makes the acoustic shadows of the ribs disappear from the entire scanned area, which is referred to as a compact B-line. The compact B-line is a common ultrasonic sign in severe TTN patients

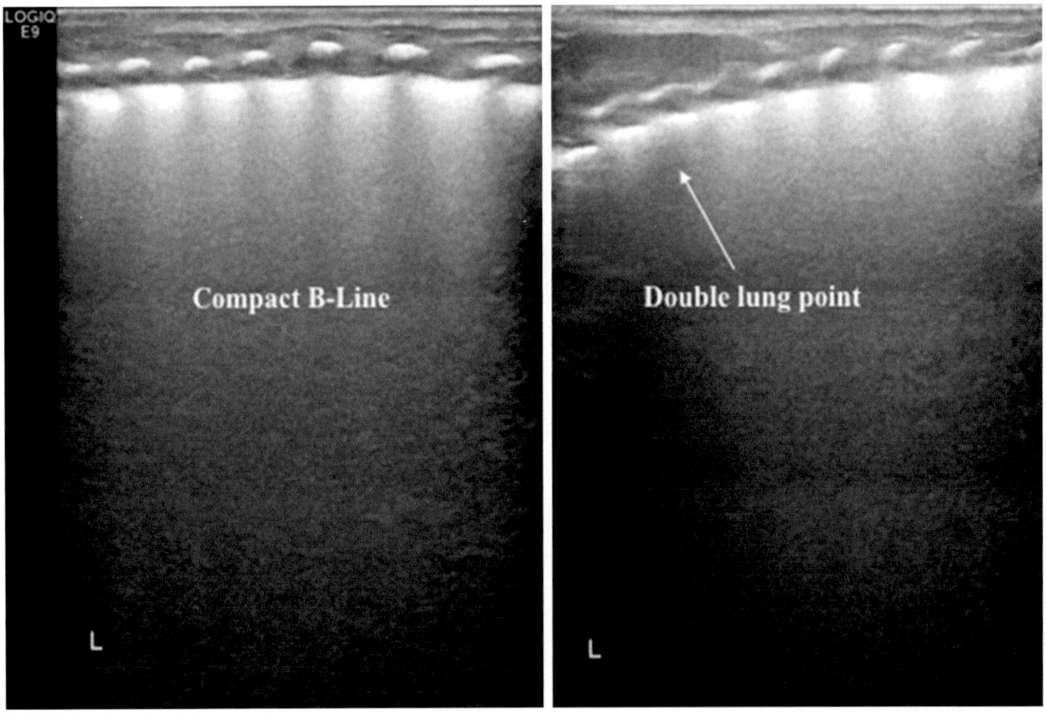

Fig. 4.9 Double lung point in the recovery stage of a severe TTN patient. A lung ultrasound shows a compact B-line in a severe TTN infant at 6 h of life (left picture) and a double lung point during the recovery stage at 42 h after birth (right picture). We confirmed that no double lung point exists in severe TTN infants but that it can be observed during recovery stages

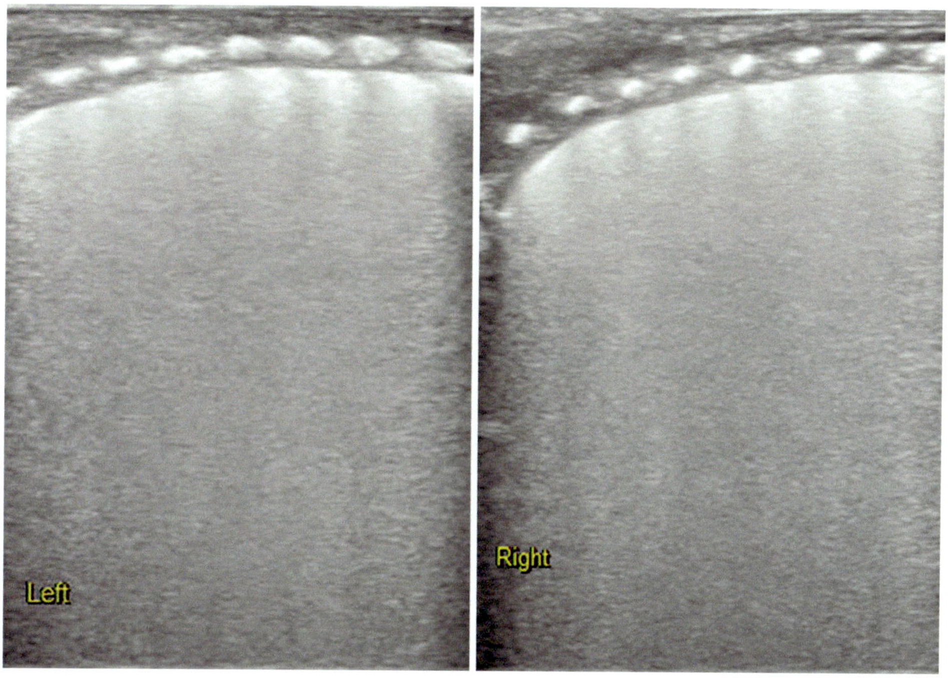

Fig. 4.10 White lung in a severe TTN infant. The infant was admitted to the hospital after suffering from dyspnea for 6 h and was diagnosed with TTN based on arterial blood gas analysis and CXR manifestation. Bilateral white lung is observed when a compact B-line exists in each lung field. Both a compact B-line and white lung are common ultrasonic signs in severe TTN. The above had a GA of 27 weeks and was delivered vaginally with a birth weight of 1020 g

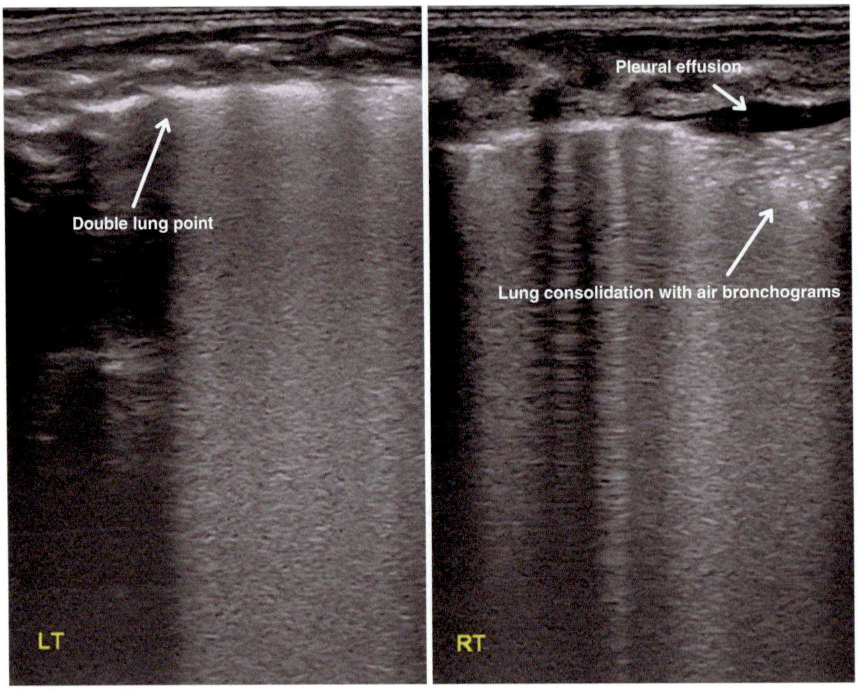

Fig. 4.11 Double lung point in RDS patient. A female infant with a gestational age of 37^{+2} weeks, who was delivered by cesarean section with a birth weight of 2850 g. The baby was admitted to the hospital due to respiratory distress 2 h after birth. The lung ultrasound found a significant double lung point in the left lung. A significant consolidation with significant air bronchograms and pleural effusion was observed in the right lung. Therefore, the patient was diagnosed with RDS and not TTN. A double lung point can also be observed in patients with other lung diseases. Therefore, this finding has non-specific manifestations of TTN

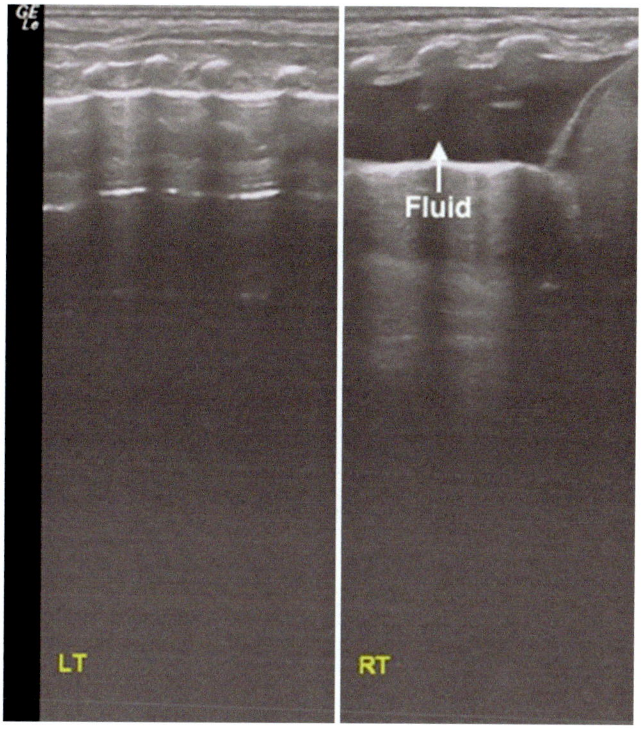

Fig. 4.12 One side of the lung can be normal in TTN patients. Edema is the major pathological lesion of TTN. However, the pathological degree in bilateral lungs could be different and could even be normal in one side of the lungs, like in this patient, who was diagnosed with TTN according to the clinical information, whose left lung was normal under ultrasound, while the right had AIS and fluid (Fig. 4.13)

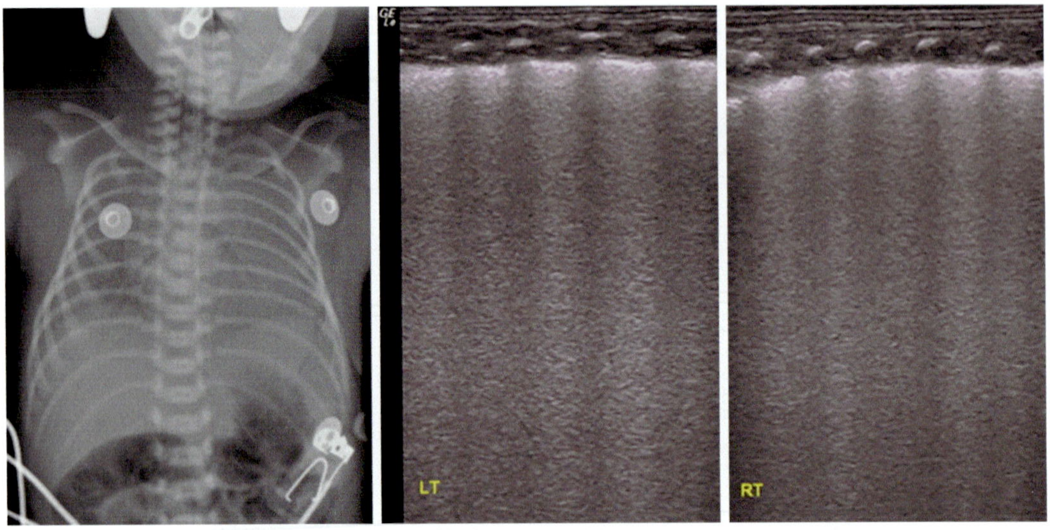

Fig. 4.13 The differential diagnosis of TTN and RDS. An infant had a gestational age of 37^{+2} weeks and was delivered by cesarean section. The birth weight of the infant was 2350 g. The baby was admitted to the hospital after suffering from birth asphyxia and dyspnea after birth for 3 h. The blood analysis showed pH 7.20, $PaCO_2$ 59 mmHg, PaO_2 37 mmHg, and $Sa0_2$ 57%, and the CRX showed that the lung penetration was significantly reduced with air bronchogram. The heart shadow was blurred, but we could still distinguish the heart contour, which indicated grade III RDS. However, the LUS showed no lung consolidation in the lungs, while AIS was present, which was lung edema. Therefore, the infant was diagnosed with TTN and not RDS (Fig. 4.14)

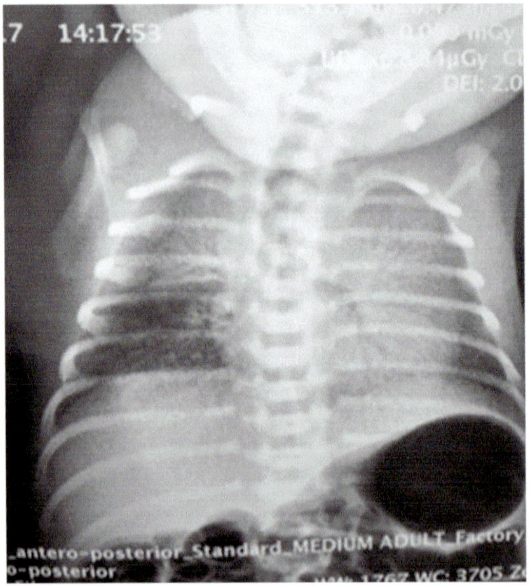

Fig. 4.14 The differential diagnosis of TTN and RDS. A baby was G_1P_1, gestational age 34 weeks, cesarean section delivery, with a birth weight of 2400 g and was admitted to our NICU due to breathing difficulties for 20 min. This baby had representative clinical manifestations, including progressive respiratory distress, tachypnea > 120/min, expiratory grunting, nasal flaring, subcostal retractions, cyanosis, etc. The arterial blood analysis showed pH 7.19, $PaCO_2$ 65 mmHg, PaO_2 51 mmHg, SaO_2 77%, and BE −17.5 mmol/L. The chest X-ray presented with nearly white lung, and the infant was diagnosed with RDS (grade IV) clinically. The lung ultrasound showed significant AIS in the bilateral lung field, irregular or coarse appearance of the pleural line, and A-line disappearance, whereas no consolidation was observed at 30 min (Fig. 4.15) or 5 h (Fig. 4.16) after birth, which indicated significant edema in the lungs. At 9 h of life, the degree of lung edema decreased (Fig. 4.17). The baby recovered almost completely at 24 h of life (Fig. 4.18). Combined with the lung ultrasound findings and the patient's clinical course, the diagnosis should have been TTN, not RDS (Fig. 4.19)

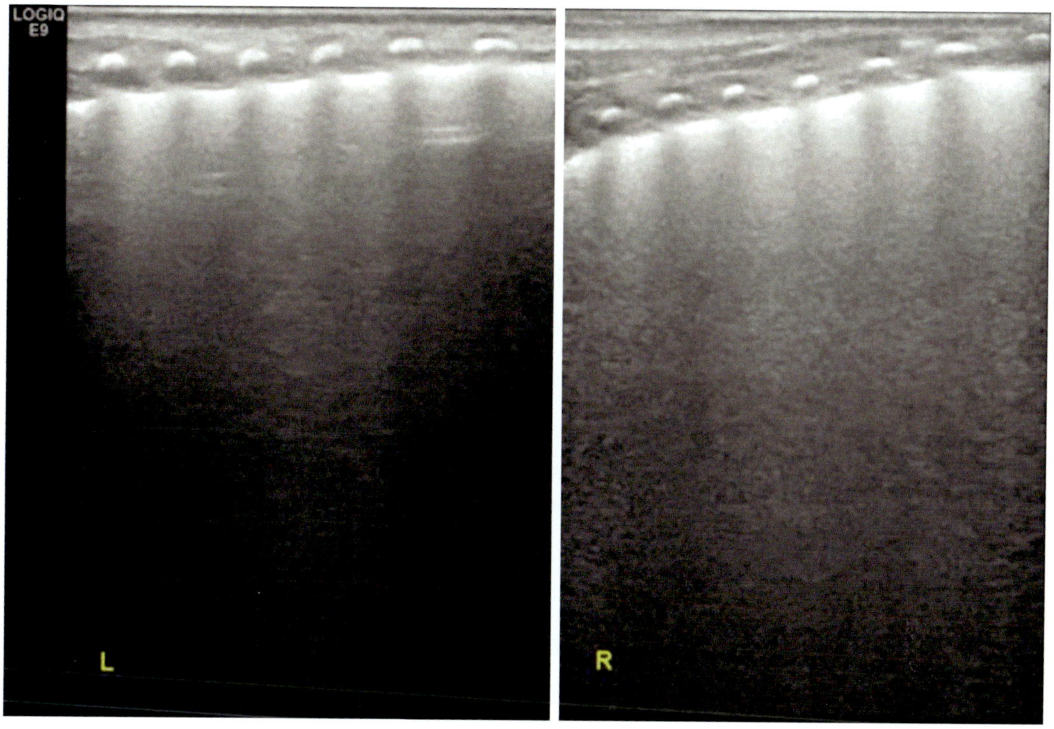

Fig. 4.15 AIS (lung edema) at 30 min after birth

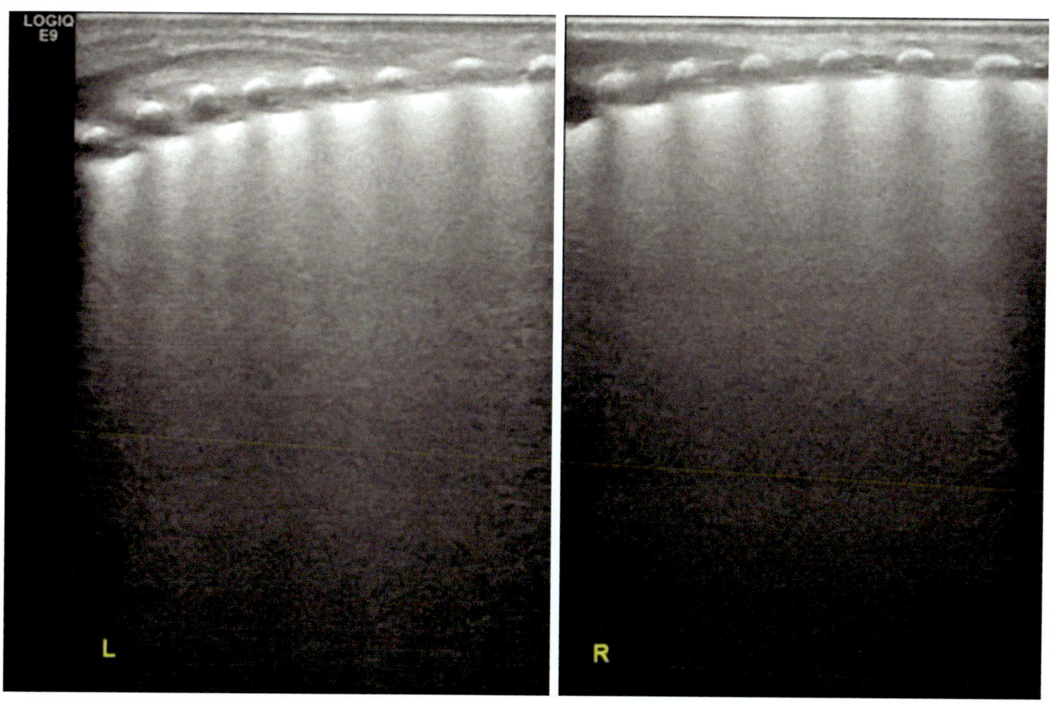

Fig. 4.16 AIS (lung edema) at 5 h after birth

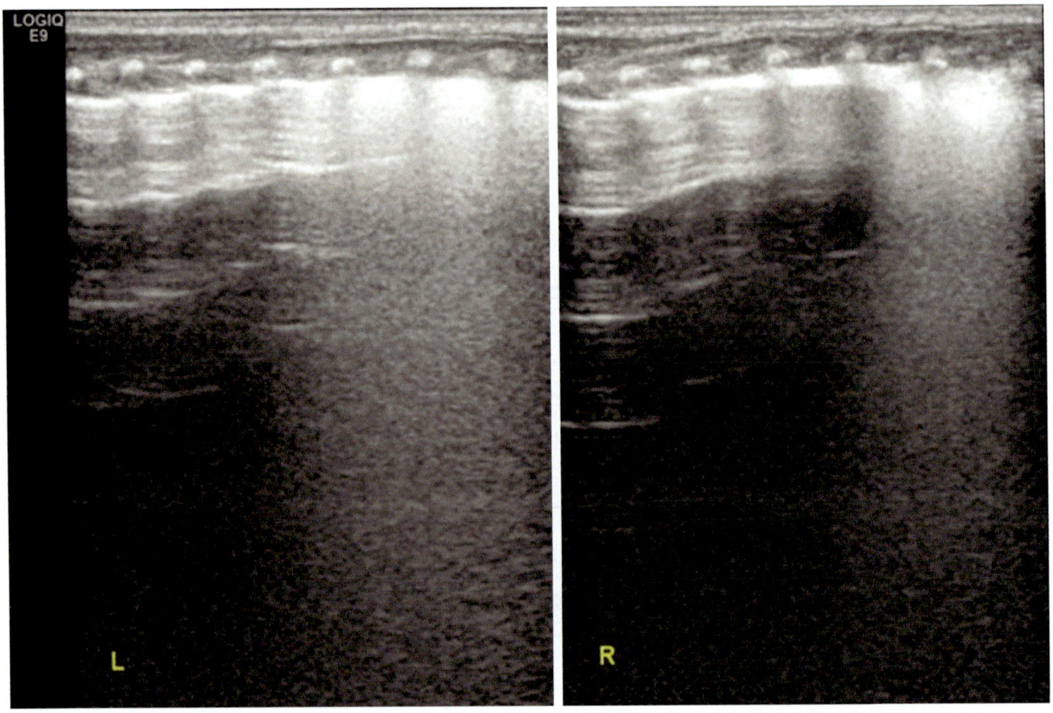

Fig. 4.17 Lung edema decreased at 9 h after birth; the pleural line and A-lines emerged in the bilateral upper lung fields

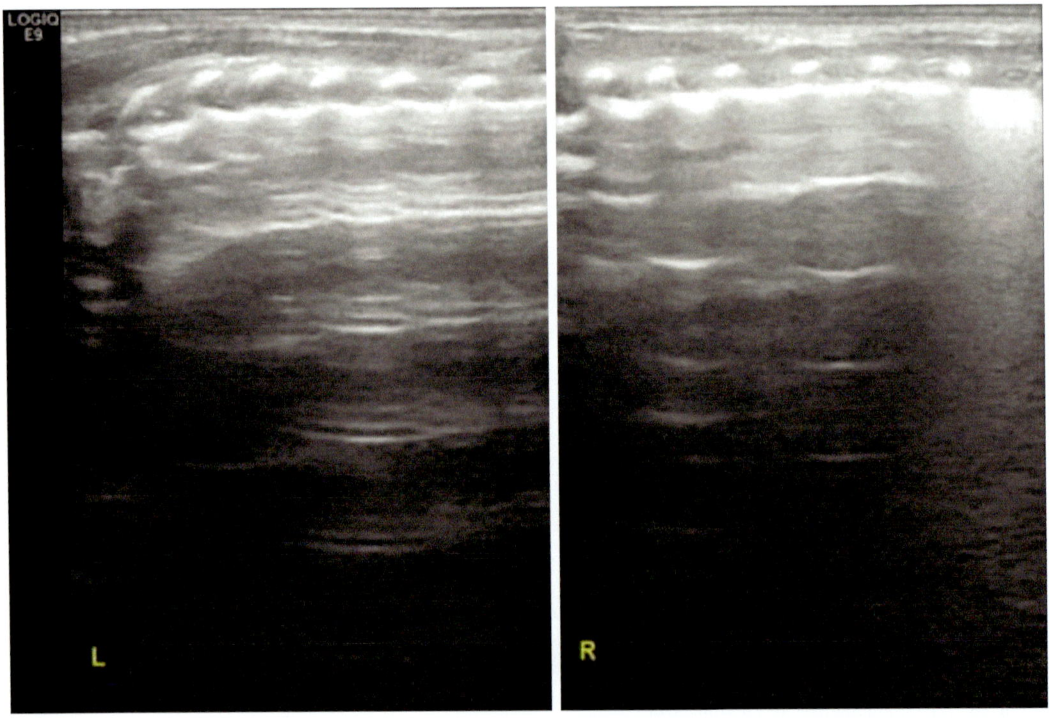

Fig. 4.18 The images returned to normal at 24 h of life, and the patient's clinical signs disappeared

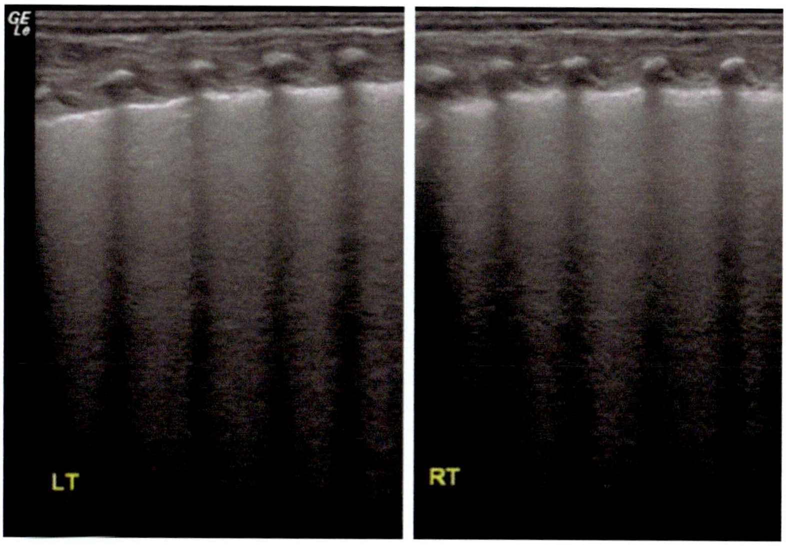

Fig. 4.19 TTN leads to RDS. An infant had a GA of 36^{+3} weeks and was delivered by cesarean section with a birth weight of 2620 g. The infant was admitted to the NICU due to dyspnea for 9 h. Lung ultrasonography showed disappearance of the pleural lines and A-lines in both lung fields. The infant was diagnosed with TTN from combined ultrasound findings, chest X-ray findings (Fig. 4.20), and clinical manifestations and was provided general care at the NICU. However, the dyspnea became severe over time, with expiratory grunting, nasal flaring, subcostal retractions, and gradually emerging cyanosis that became more significant. Reexamination of the lung ultrasound showed significant lung consolidation with air bronchograms in both lungs, indicating that RDS had developed (Fig. 4.21)

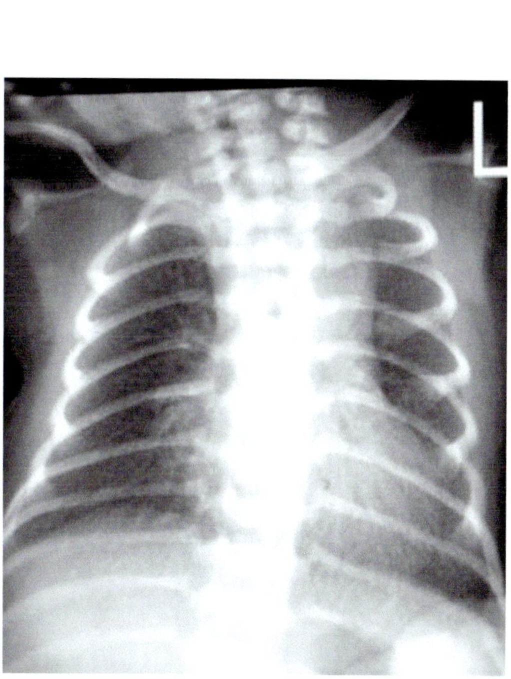

Fig. 4.20 The chest X-ray showed significant typical aerial fluid and interstitial fluid in the lung fields which are the typical chest X-ray findings in TTN patients

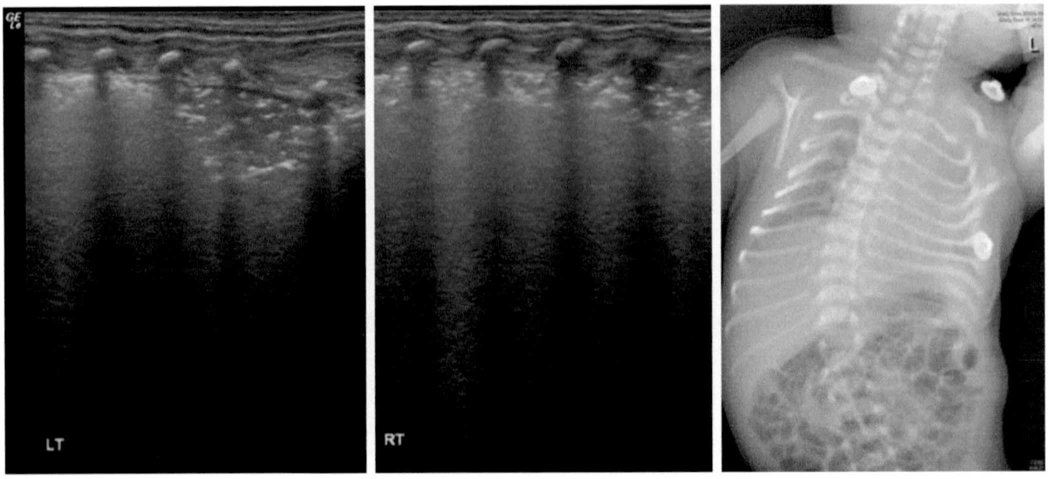

Fig. 4.21 An ultrasound showed significant lung consolidation with air bronchograms in the bilateral lungs, and the chest X-ray also confirmed RDS. This case demonstrates that TTN can lead to or develop into RDS. Thus, it is important to follow-up lung ultrasound changes, so a timely and accurate diagnosis can be made

References

1. Greenough A. Transient tachypnea of newborn. In: Greenough A, Milner AD, editors. Neonatal respiratory disorder. 2nd ed. London: CRC Press; 2003. p. 272–7.
2. Abu-Shaweesh JM. Respiratory disorder in preteen and term infants. In: Martin RJ, Fanaroff AA, Walsh MC, editors. Fanaroff and Martin's neonatal-perinatal medicine. 9th ed. Louis: Mosby; 2011. p. 1141–70.
3. Yurdakok M. Transient tachypnea of the newborn: what is new? J Matern Fetal Neonatal Med. 2010;23(S3):24–6.
4. Rocha G, Rodrigues M, Guimarães H. Respiratory distress syndrome of the preterm neonate-placenta and necropsy as witnesses. J Matern Fetal Neonatal Med. 2011;24(1):148–51.
5. Cattarossi L, Copetti R. The "double lung point": an ultrasound sign diagnostic of transient tachypnea of the newborn. Neonatology. 2007;91(3):203–9.
6. Liu J, Wang Y, Fu W, et al. The diagnosis of neonatal transient tachypnea and its differentiation from respiratory distress syndrome using lung ultrasound. Medicine. 2014a;93(27):e197.
7. Liu J, Chen XX, Li XW, et al. Lung ultrasonography to diagnose transient tachypnea of the newborn. Chest. 2016;149(5):1269–75.
8. Liu J, Cao HY, Wang HW, et al. The role of lung ultrasound in diagnosis of respiratory distress syndrome in newborn infants. Iran J Pediatr. 2014b;24(2):147–54.

Meconium Aspiration Syndrome of the Newborn

5

Jing Liu

5.1 Meconium Aspiration Syndrome

Meconium aspiration syndrome (MAS) occurs in fetuses that absorb meconium-stained amniotic fluid in the uterus or during delivery, causing the newborns to experience the main clinical manifestation of respiratory distress after birth. MAS is common in term infants or post-term infants. MAS is a serious lung disease; 10–20% of these patients will experience pneumothorax, and 5–10% of the patients will die.

The incidence of meconium staining of the amniotic fluid (MSAF) increases with gestational age. For example, the overall incidence of MSAF is approximately 12%, while the incidence is ≥30% at gestational ages of >42 weeks, <2% at gestational ages of <37 weeks, and rare at gestational ages of <34 weeks [1, 2]. Meconium excretion is a naturally occurring sign of the development of the gastrointestinal tract. For fetuses with mature nervous systems, umbilical cord compression might cause transient parasympathetic excitement and ensuing meconium excretion. Fetal distress might also trigger meconium excretion. When spontaneous breathing after birth begins, newborns might inhale meconium granules into the distal airways. Should a large amount of thick meconium be inhaled, the newborn might develop severe difficulty breathing within hours of birth, which might manifest as cyanosis, nasal flaring, signs of three depressions and shortness of breath, and expiratory groaning; in severe cases, the baby might die before birth or shortly after birth. This condition is called meconium aspiration syndrome (MAS) [3]. MAS is a serious lung disease accounting for approximately 10% of all cases of respiratory failure; 10–20% of these patients will experience pneumothorax, with a 39% mortality rate in developing and newly industrialized countries [3]. Early diagnosis and early treatment are important for improving the prognosis. Historically, MAS has been mainly diagnosed based on medical history, clinical manifestations, and chest X-ray, and ultrasonography has not been used as a diagnostic tool [4–6]. Recently, ultrasound has been used for MAS diagnosis successfully and accurately.

5.1.1 Etiology and Pathogenesis

1. Meconium discharge: The discharge of meconium induces meconium-stained amniotic fluid (MSAF). The incidence rate is related

Electronic Supplementary Material The online version of this chapter (https://doi.org/10.1007/978-94-024-1549-0_5) contains supplementary material, which is available to authorized users.

J. Liu
Department of Neonatology and NICU,
Beijing Chaoyang District Maternal and Child Health Care Hospital, Beijing, China

J. Liu et al. (eds.), *Neonatal Lung Ultrasonography*, https://doi.org/10.1007/978-94-024-1549-0_5

with gestational age; the higher the gestational age, the greater the incidence rate. The overall incidence rate is approximately 12%; for those with a gestational age >42 weeks, the incidence rate can reach more than 30%; for those with a gestational age <37 weeks, the incidence rate is less than 2%; and for those with a gestational age <34 weeks, very few will experience MAS.

Meconium excretion is a naturally occurring sign of the development of the gastrointestinal tract; for fetuses with a mature nervous system, umbilical cord compression can cause temporary parasympathetic nervous excitement and cause meconium discharge, and fetal intrauterine distress can trigger the discharge of meconium. It is generally accepted that meconium-stained amniotic fluid is associated with chronic intrauterine hypoxia, fetal acidosis, and a poor prognosis, and MSAF with an abnormal fetal heart rate is a sign of fetal distress and the occurrence of perinatal complications. By observing the color of the meconium-stained amniotic fluid, the time of meconium discharge or fetal distress occurrence can be broadly speculated; a color of yellow indicates old meconium, and a color of green often indicates recently discharged meconium.

2. Meconium aspiration: Under normal circumstances, the secretion of fetal lung fluid is large, and the liquid in the airway flows out from the airway into the amniotic cavity. When there is no apparent intrauterine distress, even if the amniotic fluid contains meconium, the normal fetal breathing movement will not lead to meconium inhalation, as the inhaled meconium particles are only found in the upper airways or to the main trachea without causing serious symptoms. In cases in which obvious intrauterine distress causes fetal gasping, the meconium particles can be inhaled into the small airway or the alveoli. After the fetus starts breathing on its own, especially when accompanied by wheezing, meconium particles can be inhaled into the distal airways.
3. Pathophysiology: The main manifestations are heterogeneous mechanical obstruction of the airway and chemical inflammatory reactions induced by meconium. (1) Atelectasis and emphysema: The inhalation of meconium particles into the distal airways first causes mechanical obstruction of the small airways; when the obstruction is complete, it leads to atelectasis; when the obstruction is partial, it causes a flap oxygen effect. At this time, inspiration is an active process, and the airway pressure difference produced by the thoracic cavity negative pressure effect is relatively large on inspiration, making it easy for gas to enter the lungs; expiration is a passive process, and the pressure difference is relatively small, making it difficult for the gas to be exhaled, eventually inducing alveolar gas retention so that emphysema is caused, alveolar ventilation is decreased, and CO_2 retention is introduced. In serious cases, alveoli occur, inducing the occurrence of pulmonary interstitial emphysema, mediastinal emphysema, or pneumothorax; 12–24 h after meconium aspiration, chemical inflammation and pulmonary interstitial edema are induced due to the chemical stimulation of meconium on the small airways; chemical inflammation makes pulmonary emphysema persistently present, and lung collapse is more obvious. Under the microscope, neutrophil infiltration, alveolar and airway epithelial cell necrosis, and intra-alveolar protein-like fragment accumulation are seen in the alveolar septa. The obstruction of the airway can cause the pulmonary compliance to decrease. Soluble protease, free fatty acids, phospholipids, bile salt, blood, lanugo, exfoliated cells, bilirubin, protein, cholesterol, triglycerides, and other ingredients are contained in the meconium and deactivate pulmonary surfactants, affecting the generation of SP-A and SP-B and further causing a lack of secondary pulmonary surfactants; as a result, the lung compliance further decreases, and lung collapse becomes further aggravated. (2) Normal alveoli: Part of the small airways might be meconium-free, and the alveolar ventilation-gas exchange functions will increase compensatorily. The lung changes in MAS result in heterogeneous airway obstruction, namely, the coexistence of atelectasis, emphysema, and

normal alveoli, and their proportions can decide the severity of clinical manifestations. (3) Pulmonary hypertension: Based on asphyxia and anoxia, meconium aspiration induced by atelectasis, chemical inflammatory injuries, and secondary PS deficiency further aggravates atelectasis, hypoventilation, and hypoxemia. The above factors render the pulmonary vascular pressure incapable of decreasing due to maladaptation to the dramatic changes in the environment after birth, and the pressure increases, eventually resulting in persistent pulmonary hypertension of the newborn (PPHN); approximately one-third of infants experience PPHN of varying degrees. In addition, intrauterine chronic hypoxia induces pulmonary arterial dysplasia, which means the vascular smooth muscle extends to the normal non-muscularized intra-acinar arterioles, resulting in the narrowing of small vessel lumens and an increase of pulmonary vascular resistance, which is also involved in the pathogenesis of PPHN. (4) Secondary pulmonary surfactant deficiency: The mechanical irritation of meconium particles and the chemical stimulation of bile salts in meconium can directly induce alveolar type II cell damage, and hypoxia and acidosis can inhibit pulmonary surfactant synthesis and destroy its functions, leading to secondary pulmonary surfactant deficiency. (5) Hypoxemia and mixed acidosis: The combined effect of the above factors results in severe dysfunction of ventilation and air exchange and induces serious hypoxemia and mixed acidosis; in severe cases, severe respiratory failure, pulmonary edema, and pulmonary bleeding occur.

5.1.2 Clinical Manifestations

1. Meconium-stained amniotic fluid—MAS is common in postmature infants, and meconium-stained amniotic fluid is a prerequisite for the diagnosis of MAS as follows: (1) visible amniotic fluid mixed with meconium during childbirth; (2) visible severe jaundice of the skin, nails, umbilical cord, and other parts after the birth of infants; (3) visible or suckable meconium or meconium-stained fluid in infants' oral and nasal cavity; and (4) in tracheal intubation when meconium particles can be sucked from the glottis or trachea, the diagnosis can be confirmed.
2. Respiratory system manifestations: The severity of symptoms is associated with the nature of the aspirated amniotic fluid (suspension or massive meconium) and the amount. Those with a small inhalation volume and homogeneously mixed amniotic fluid can be asymptomatic or might experience mild symptoms; as for those with a large inhalation of sticky meconium volume, a dead fetus can be induced, or they might die soon after birth. Usually, dyspnea appears within a few hours after birth, with the manifestations of cyanosis, nasal flaring, retractions and significant shortness of breath, and shallow and fast respiration; only a minority of patients experience grunting. The manifestation of early respiratory abnormalities is induced by the inhalation of pulmonary meconium into the body due to the delay of lung field cleaning. Lung hyperinflation can cause chest anteroposterior diameter enlargement, resulting in a barrel chest; rales can be heard through lung auscultation. At 12–24 h after birth, as the meconium granules are further aspirated into the distal airways, the above symptoms and signs become more obvious. Because the inhaled meconium particles are ultimately subject to phagocytic clearance, the dyspnea in infants can last for several days and even several weeks. If symptoms are relieved within 24–48 h after birth, it can be induced by lung fluid clearance delay (viz., TTN) instead of MAS.
3. PPHN manifestations: Severe cyanosis is the main manifestation, which is characterized by a high concentration (>60%) of oxygen, cyanosis incapable of being alleviated, and aggravation with crying, feeding, and restlessness; the degree of cyanosis and pulmonary physical signs is not parallel (i.e., severe cyanosis and light pulmonary signs). In severe cases, heart failure and shock occur. A systolic murmur can be heard in

the second rib of the chest bone left margin. The following tests are helpful in the differentiation of the causes of cyanosis. (1) Hyperoxia test: inhale pure oxygen for 15 min; if the arterial oxygen partial pressure (PaO_2) or transcutaneous oxygen saturation ($TcSO_2$) increases significantly compared with baseline, pulmonary parenchymal lesions are indicated; if there is no significant change, PPHN or cyanotic congenital heart disease is indicated. (2) Arterial catheterization before and after blood oxygen difference test: a comparison is made in terms of PaO_2 and $TcSO_2$ before (right radial artery or temporal artery) and after (left radial or lower extremity arteries) arterial catheterization; in case the catheterization before/after PaO_2 difference >2 kPa (15 mmHg) or $TcSO_2$ >4%, it is suggested that a right-to-left shunt is present at the level of arterial catheterization (but without a difference, PPHN cannot be ruled out because the right-to-left shunt at the foramen ovale has no influence). (3) Hyperoxia-hyperventilation test: perform endotracheal intubation ventilation with pure oxygen for 10–15 min at the frequency of 60–80 times/min, making the carbon dioxide partial pressure ($PaCO_2$) decrease and blood pH value increase; if the PaO_2 >4 kPa or $TcSO_2$ >8% when compared with the values before ventilation, it is suggested that PPHN is present and no such change is observed in cyanotic congenital heart disease.

4. Other manifestations: Severe MAS might be complicated by polycythemia, hypoglycemia, hypocalcemia, hypoxic-ischemic encephalopathy, multiple organ dysfunction and pulmonary bleeding, etc.

5.1.3 Common Used Examinations

1. Laboratory tests: Arterial blood gas analysis shows that pH value decreases, PaO_2 decreases, and $PaCO_2$ increases with the manifestations of hypoxemia and hypercapnia, with severe mixed acidosis. Other examinations, such as blood, blood sugar, blood calcium, blood biochemical tests, and if necessary, endotracheal aspirate culture or blood culture, might be needed.
2. Chest X-ray examination: A chest X-ray is of important significance in the diagnosis of MAS; inhaled meconium usually reaches the alveoli 4 h after birth, and then a chest X-ray can have special manifestations. The X-ray findings of approximately 85% of infants with MAS are the most obvious 48 h after birth, but the chest X-ray findings of approximately 70% of infants with MAS might not be consistent with the clinical manifestations, and the main manifestations are the enhanced permeability of both lungs accompanied with segmental or small lobular atelectasis and only the presence of diffuse infiltration shadows or concurrent mediastinal emphysema and pneumothorax. According to the X-ray manifestations, MSA can be classified as follows: (1) Mild: the pulmonary markings become thickened, the pulmonary emphysema is mild, the diaphragmatic muscles drop mildly, and the cardiac shadow is normal, indicating that relatively sparse meconium is aspirated. (2) Moderate: the lung field has coarse particles or lamellar lumps with increased density and cottony cloud-shaped shadows or segmental atelectasis, accompanied by mildly translucent cystic emphysema and a slightly small size of heart shadows. (3) Severe: in addition to the above moderate manifestations, the diseases are also accompanied by interstitial emphysema, pneumomediastinum, pneumothorax, or other gas leakage phenomena.

5.1.4 Differential Diagnosis

1. Respiratory distress syndrome of newborn: It frequently occurs to premature infants; lack of pulmonary surfactant leads to progressive atelectasis with rapid-onset, progressive dyspnea, cyanosis, retraction and expiratory groaning; the X-ray chest film indicates that the brightness of the two lungs declines generally, and an air bronchogram can be seen. The details are shown in relevant chapters.
2. Amniotic fluid aspiration pneumonia: Simple amniotic fluid is easier to be absorbed, and symptoms are mild with fewer complications.

5.1.5 Treatment

1. Endotracheal meconium aspiration: For infants with serious conditions and who were just born, endotracheal intubation should be performed for endotracheal aspiration to minimize the complete absorption of the airway meconium and to help relieve the conditions and prevent the occurrence of PPHN. Animal experiments show that meconium can still be sucked from the airway for 4 h after the meconium is aspirated into the airway.
2. Symptomatic treatment is as follows: Correct hypoxia, acidosis, and shock; ensure that the airway is smooth; as for those with respiratory failure, provide mechanical ventilation for therapy; pay attention to keeping the newborn warm, providing enough calories, ensuring proper electrolyte balance, and limiting fluid properly; complement exogenous pulmonary surfactant.
3. PPHN treatment: Alkalize the blood, give high-frequency ventilation (>50–60 times/min), and maintain the blood PH value of 7.45–7.55; administer vasoactive drugs to reduce pulmonary artery pressure, increase systemic circulation pressure, give nitric oxide inhalation for treatment, and for the those with conditions, use extracorporeal membrane oxygenator for treatment.
4. An echocardiogram can be used to assist with ruling out congenital heart disease, to determine the pulmonary artery pressure, and to ascertain if a right-to-left shunt is present.

5.2 Ultrasound Diagnosis of Meconium Aspiration Syndrome

A previous study described the lung ultrasound signs in six patients with MAS; these signs included the following [7]: (1) coalescent or sparse B-pattern, (2) consolidations, (3) atelectasis, and (4) bronchograms. The authors reported that the lung ultrasound images corresponded well with the X-ray findings. This present study demonstrated that lung ultrasonography was accurate and reliable for the diagnosis of MAS. Based on the results of our study, the main ultrasonographic characteristics of MAS were as follows [8]: (1) Lung consolidation with air bronchogram was found in all patients, usually with a large consolidation area with irregular edges. According to this present study, the signs of lung consolidation with irregular margins on ultrasonography had 100% sensitivity and 100% specificity for diagnosing MAS; (2) there was variation in the nature and extent of pulmonary lesions between lungs or in the same lung. The area of lung consolidation varied between the lungs, and different sizes of consolidated areas were present in the same lung. A large consolidation was often seen in severely affected patients, whereas small consolidations and confluent B-lines were often seen in patients with less severe MAS; (3) atelectasis was found in a few (16.2%) severe cases in our present study. Lung pulse was found in severe cases (8.5%). There was an absence of lung sliding in all patients with atelectasis; (4) pleural line anomalies were seen, including disappearance of the pleural line or thickened and blurred pleural lines in the area of lesions; (5) disappearance of the A-line was observed; (6) the B-line or AIS was observed in the non-consolidation area; (7) pleural effusion was found in 13.7% of patients in this present study. However, these ultrasonographic findings are also observed in lung diseases such as RDS, pneumonia, and atelectasis, so they are not specific to MAS [9–11]. In particular, large areas of pulmonary consolidation with irregular edges are also observed on lung ultrasonography in cases of pneumonia [11], which is useful for differentiating between MAS and other diseases. MAS and pneumonia can be differentiated because varying degrees of pulmonary consolidation are usually observed in both lungs in MAS but only in one lung in pneumonia (Figs. 5.1, 5.2, 5.3, 5.4, 5.5, 5.6, 5.7, 5.8, and 5.9).

We stated that all the pictures or ultrasound images included in the chapter were taken from the Army General Hospital of the Chinese PLA and Beijing Chaoyang District Maternal and Child Healthcare Hospital and the related studies were approved by both the committee of the Army General Hospital and Chaoyang District Maternal and Child Healthcare Hospital.

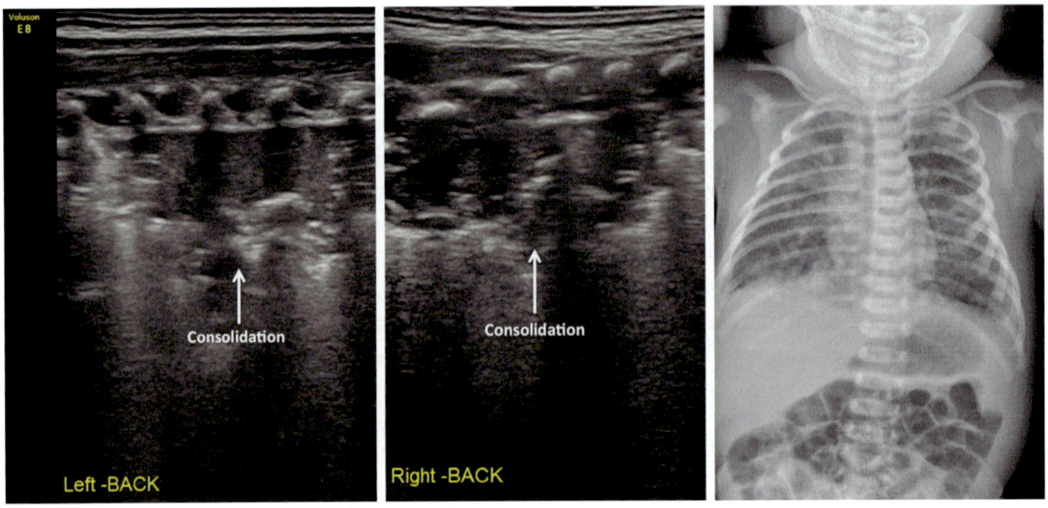

Fig. 5.1 Lung ultrasonographic findings in MAS. G1P1, 41 weeks of gestation, birth weight 3330 g. MSAF, asphyxia at birth, difficulty breathing after resuscitation. Lung ultrasonography showed large areas of pulmonary consolidation with air bronchogram and irregular edges in the lungs. The pleural line was abnormal, and the A-line disappeared in the consolidation area. Chest X-ray showed patchy and cloudy shadows that were consistent with MAS

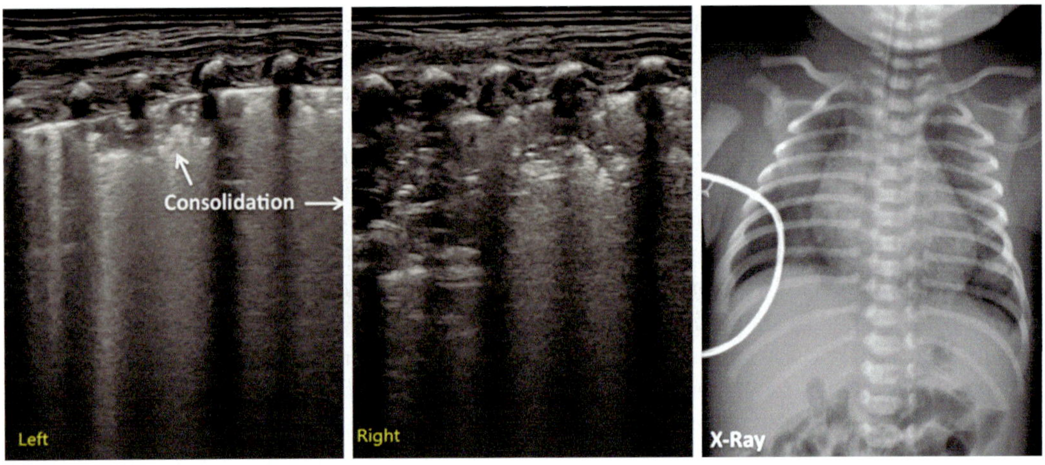

Fig. 5.2 Lung ultrasonographic findings in MAS. G_3P1, 39^{+6} weeks of gestation, vaginal birth, birth weight 3350 g. Fetal distress, MSAF, decreased amniotic fluid. At 37 weeks, the umbilical cord was wrapped twice around the feet and was twisted. Apgar scores at birth were 7, 10, and 10 points at 1, 5, and 10 min, respectively, and the heart rate was <80 bpm. There was no premature rupture of fetal membranes according to the patient's family. The newborn had difficulty breathing after birth. The patient was transferred to our hospital with endotracheal intubation and positive pressure ventilation. Lung ultrasonography showed large areas of pulmonary consolidation with irregular edges in the lungs, especially in the right lung

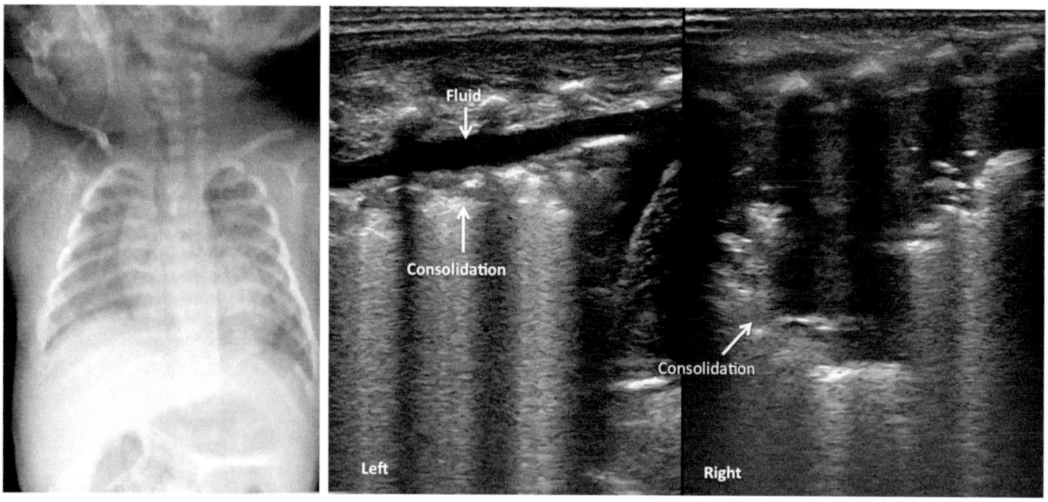

Fig. 5.3 Consolidation with pleural effusion in MAS patient. In addition to consolidation, MAS can also have one or two sides of pleural effusion. This patient was diagnosed with MAS according to clinical information and chest X-ray manifestations, and the lung ultrasound showed mild consolidation with little fluid in the left lung and a large area of consolidation in the right lung field

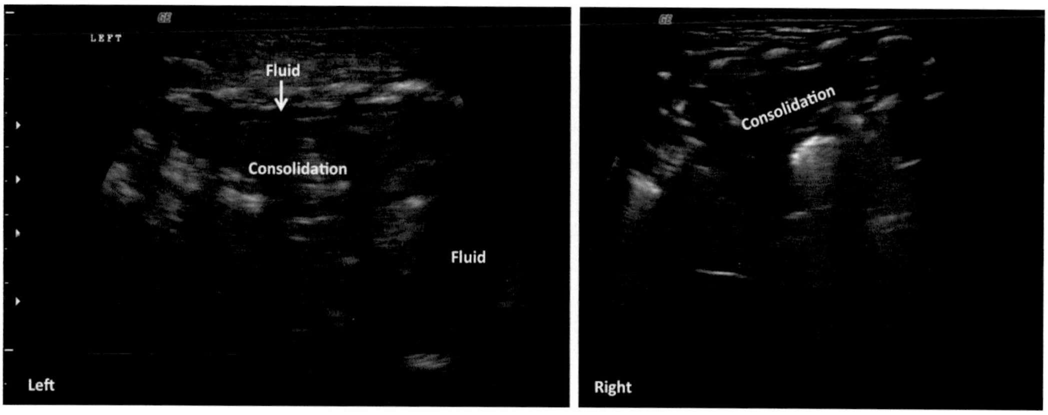

Fig. 5.4 Consolidation with pleural effusion in MAS patient. As in Fig. 5.3, in addition to significant consolidation in the lungs (more severe in left lung field, which has already lead to atelectasis), the lung ultrasound showed severe pleural effusion in the left chest

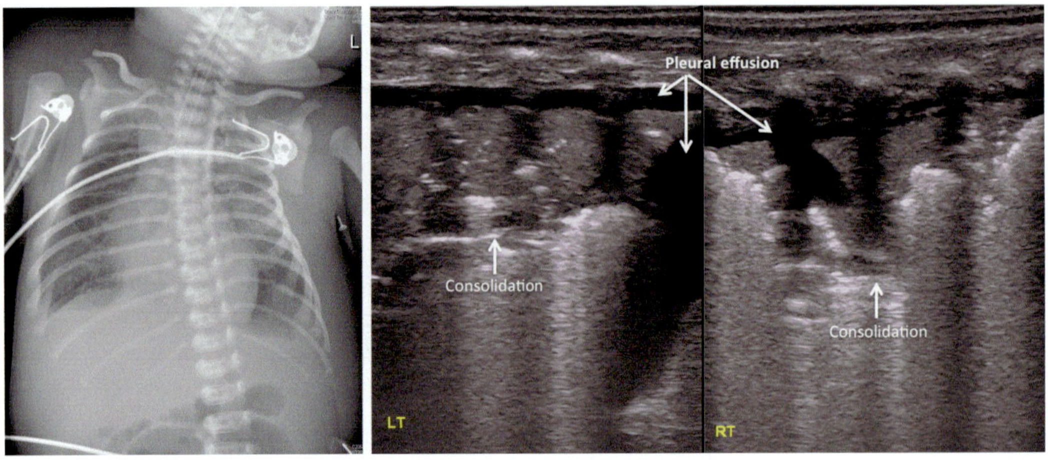

Fig. 5.5 Consolidation, pleural effusion, and lung pulse in MAS patient. The baby was G_1P_1, 41 weeks of gestation, birth weight 3330 g. MSAF, asphyxia at birth, difficulty breathing after resuscitation. X-ray showed patchy and cloudy shadows that were consistent with MAS and blunting of the costal diaphragm angle. Lung ultrasonography showed large areas of lung consolidation with air bronchogram and irregular edges in the lungs and significantly pleural effusions in both sides of the chest. The pleural line was abnormal, and the A-line disappeared. A significant lung pulse could be seen on real-time ultrasound (Video 5.1)

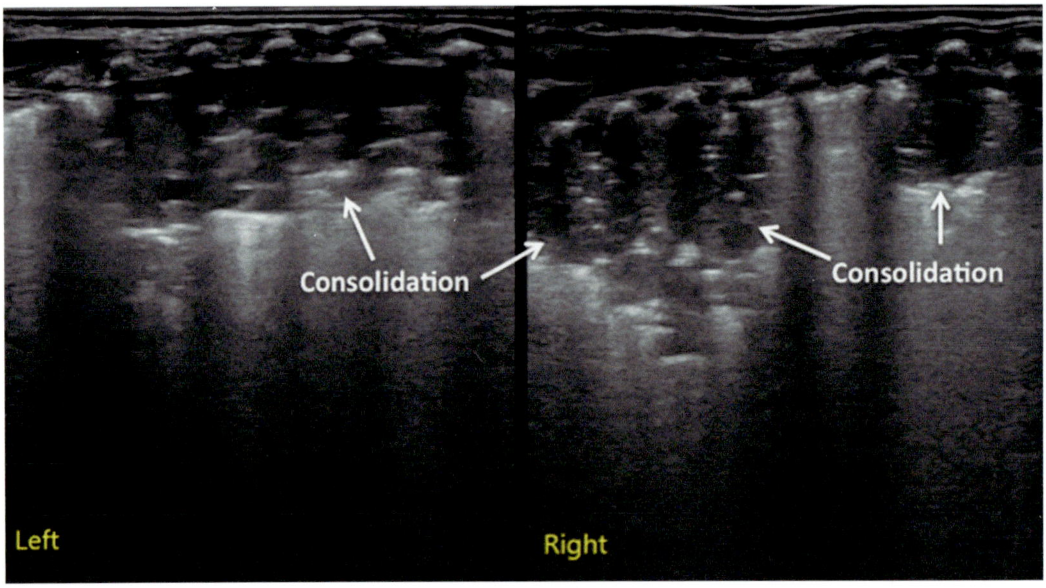

Fig. 5.6 Lung ultrasonographic findings in MAS. MAS in a full-term newborn infant. Large areas of pulmonary consolidation with air bronchogram shown on lung ultrasonography; two consolidation areas of different sizes are shown in the right lung, the pleural line blurred or disappeared, and the A-line disappeared

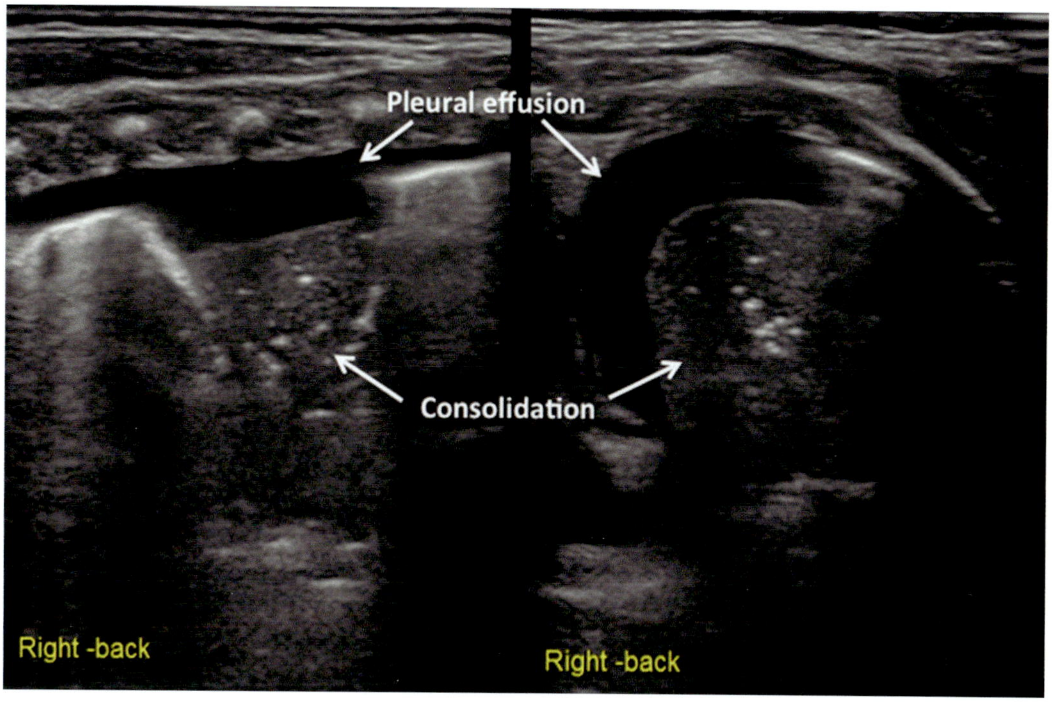

Fig. 5.7 Lung ultrasonographic findings in MAS. MAS patient. Lung ultrasonography showed large areas of pulmonary consolidation with air bronchogram and clear edges in the right lung that were consistent with atelectasis. The pleural line blurred or disappeared, and the A-line disappeared. Apparent hyperechoic fluid-filled areas were present in the chest, suggesting pleural effusion (left, the handpiece was perpendicular to the ribs; right, the handpiece was parallel to the ribs)

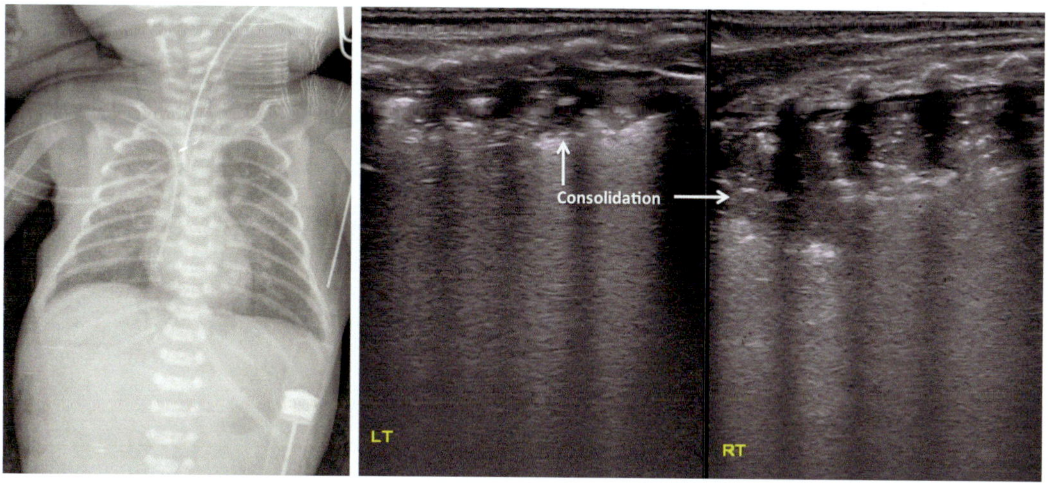

Fig. 5.8 MAS in premature infant. Gestational age of 32 weeks, C-section due to intrauterine distress, meconium-stained amniotic fluid. Severe dyspnea occurred after birth. After admission and in combination of the history, clinical manifestations, and chest X-ray changes, the diagnosis of MAS was made. Lung ultrasound showed consolidation areas in the bilateral lung fields, more significantly in the right lung field, and a small amount of pleural effusion could be seen also in the lungs. The pleural lines and A-lines of both lungs disappeared

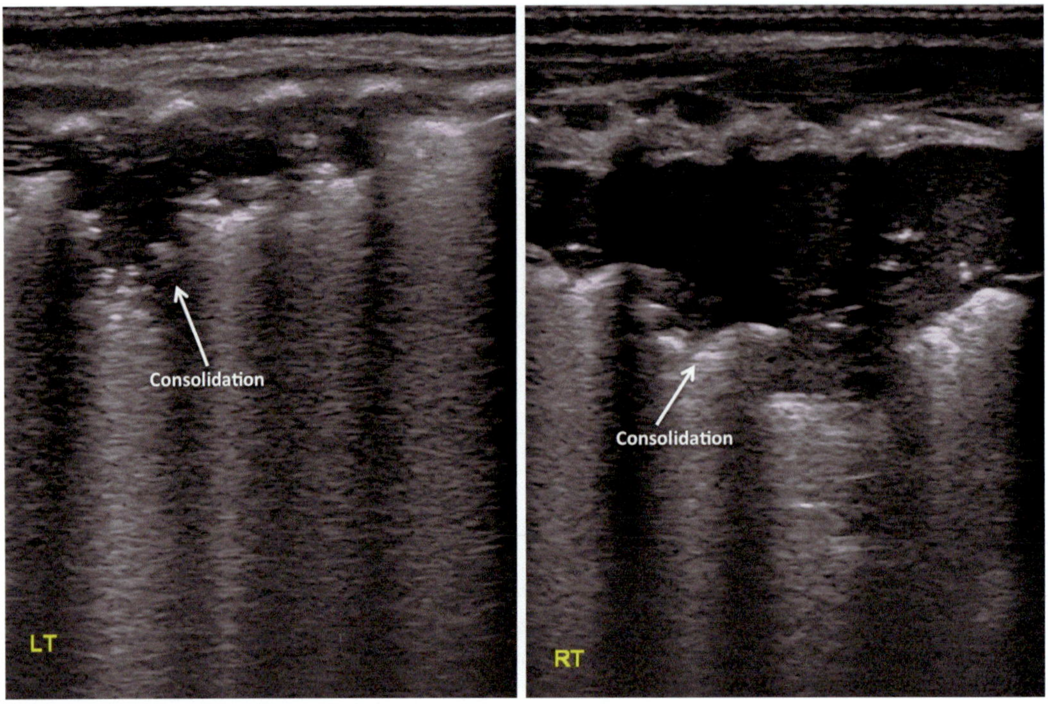

Fig. 5.9 MAS in premature infant. A gestational age of 31 weeks baby diagnosed with MAS. Ultrasound found significant consolidation in the lungs, more severe in the right lung, resulting in atelectasis. The pleural lines disappeared in the area of consolidations, and the A-lines disappeared in both sides of the lungs

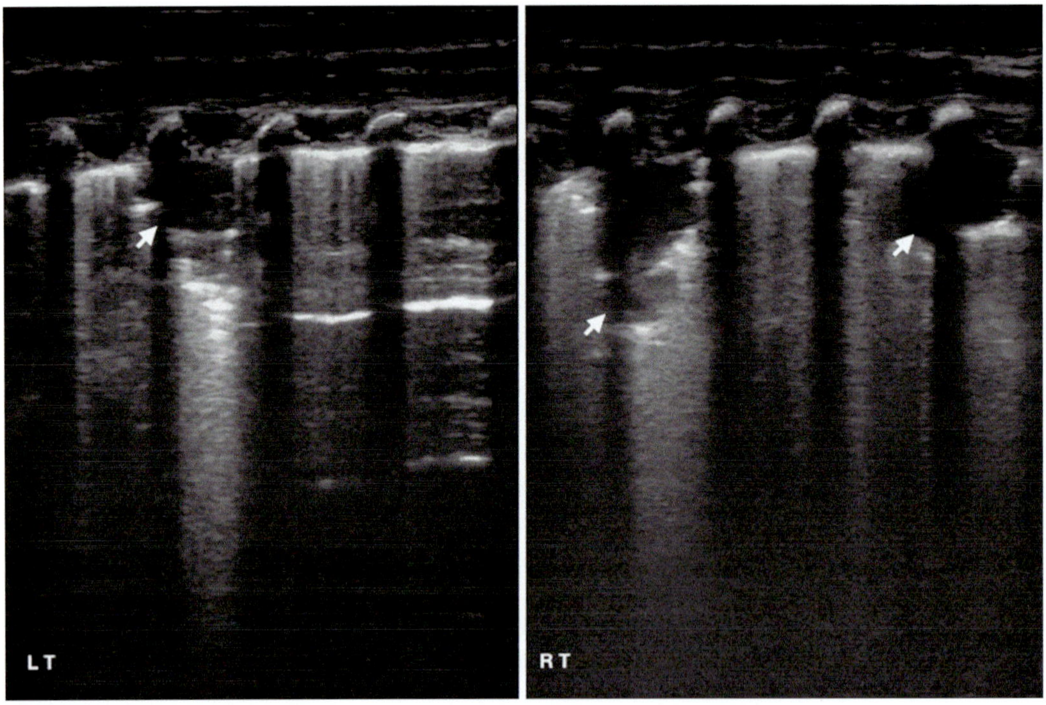

Fig. 5.10 Mild MAS. A mild MAS patient. Lung ultrasound showed small consolidation involved in one intercostal space in the left lung field and two e intercostal space in the right lung field (arrow), while the others remain normal or presented as confluent B-line

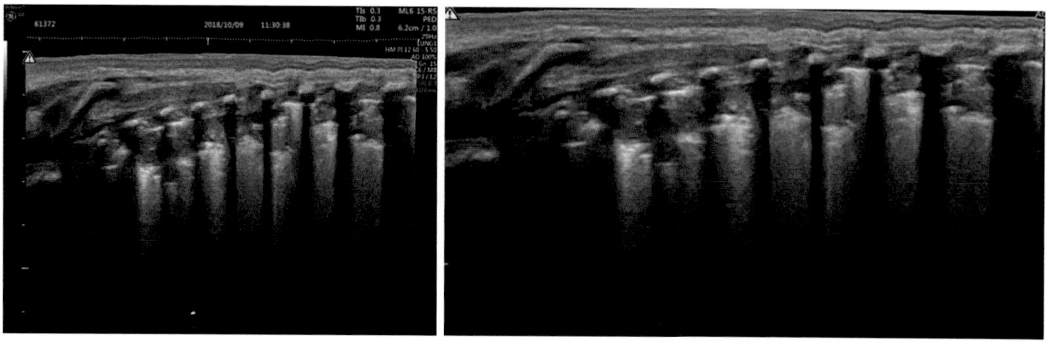

Fig. 5.11 Figure legends (volume panorama mode). Mild MAS patient. Ultrasound (volume panorama) showed small subpleural consolidation within each intercostal space in the right lung field, as well as the pleural line and A-lines disappearance

Lung ultrasonography appears to be an accurate, reliable, simple, and noninvasive technology for the diagnosis of MAS and can be performed at the bedside. Moreover, lung ultrasonography can be readily performed and is suitable for dynamic monitoring, and it can provide timely and valuable medical information when clinicians need to determine the causes of sudden changes in the patient's condition. It is very easy to distinguish MAS from other lung diseases, such as transient tachypnea of the newborn, RDS, pneumonia, and atelectasis, by using lung ultrasound.

References

1. Parker TA, Kinsella JP. Meconium aspiration syndrome. In: Gleason CA, Devaskar SU, editors. Avery's diseases of the newborn. 9th ed. Philadelphia: Elsevier Saunders; 2012. p. 652–3.
2. Abu-Shaweesh JM. Meconium aspiration syndrome. In: Martin RJ, Fanaroff AA, Walsh MC, editors. Fanaroff and Martin's neonatal-perinatal medicine. 9th ed. Louis: Elsevier Mosby; 2011. p. 1157–60.
3. Swarnam K, Soraisham AS, Sivanandan S. Advances in the management of meconium aspiration syndrome. Int J Pediatr. 2012;2012:359571.
4. van Yerland Y, de Beaufort AJ. Why does meconium cause meconium aspiration syndrome? Current concepts of MAS pathophysiology. Early Hum Dev. 2009;85:617–20.
5. Dargaville PA, Copnell B, Australian and New Zealand Neonatal Network. The epidemiology of meconium aspiration syndrome: incidence, risk factors, therapies, and outcome. Pediatrics. 2006;117:1712–21.
6. Xu H, Hofmeyr J, Roy C, et al. Intrapartum amnioinfusion for meconium-stained amniotic fluid: a systematic review of randomised controlled trials. BJOG. 2007;114:383–90.
7. Piastra M, Yousef N, Brat R, et al. Lung ultrasound findings in meconium aspiration syndrome. Early Hum Dev. 2014;90(Suppl 2):S41–3.
8. Liu J, Cao HY, Fu W. Lung ultrasonography to diagnose meconium aspiration syndrome of the newborn. J Int Med Res. 2016;44(6):1534–42.
9. Liu J, Cao HY, Wang HW, et al. The role of lung ultrasound in diagnosis of respiratory distress syndrome in newborn infants. Iran J Pediatr. 2014;24:147–54.
10. Liu J, Chen SW, Liu F, et al. The diagnosis of neonatal pulmonary atelectasis using lung ultrasonography. Chest. 2015;147:1013–9.
11. Liu J, Liu F, Liu Y, et al. Lung ultrasonography for the diagnosis of severe neonatal pneumonia. Chest. 2014;146:383–8.

6 Infectious Pneumonia of the Newborn

Jing Liu

6.1 Infectious Pneumonia

Infectious pneumonia is the most common disease in newborns and is also an important cause of neonatal death. According to statistics, infectious pneumonia accounts for more than 1/3 of the total number of newborn hospitalizations, and the number of deaths due to infectious pneumonia accounts for more than 1/4 of the total number of deaths in newborns and for more than 1/5 of neonate autopsy cases [1, 2]. Infection can occur inside the uterus, during delivery or after birth, and prenatal pathogens can infect fetuses through the blood circulating through the placenta and amniotic membrane, or pathogenic bacteria can ascend to infect fetuses due to the premature rupture of membranes. In intrapartum cases, infection is induced because fetuses are contaminated with amniotic fluid or maternal cervical secretions during delivery [2, 3]. Postpartum infection primarily occurs through the respiratory tract, through the blood or through an iatrogenic route. Common pathogens include *Escherichia coli*, *Staphylococcus aureus*, viruses (such as cytomegalovirus, herpes simplex virus, rubella virus, *Coxsackie virus*, and chicken pox virus), *Klebsiella*, *Listeria*, *Mycoplasma*, and *Chlamydia* [2, 3].

6.1.1 Etiologic Factors

1. Intrauterine infection: Primary intrauterine infection pathogens include group B β-hemolytic streptococcus, pneumoniae bacteria, *Escherichia coli*, *Klebsiella pneumoniae*, *Bacillus proteus*, cytomegalovirus, rubella virus, and herpes simplex virus. (1) Maternal infection: when the mother suffers from sepsis, viremia, or viremia and chorioamnionitis, pathogens can enter the fetal circulatory system from the mother, through placental barriers, and reach the fetal lungs to induce fetal infectious pneumonia. (2) Premature rupture of membrane (PROM): the PROM and infections in fetuses and neonates are closely related. It was previously thought that the when PROM was longer, the fetal and neonatal infection rates would be increased and the degree of infection would be more serious. However, our recent survey shows that the PROM duration and incidence of neonatal infections have no correlation. For neonates with a PROM time ≤24 h, the positive blood culture rate was 7.7%; with a PROM time of

Electronic Supplementary Material The online version of this chapter (https://doi.org/10.1007/978-94-024-1549-0_6) contains supplementary material, which is available to authorized users.

J. Liu
Department of Neonatology and NICU,
Beijing Chaoyang District Maternal and Child Health Care Hospital, Beijing, China

J. Liu et al. (eds.), *Neonatal Lung Ultrasonography*, https://doi.org/10.1007/978-94-024-1549-0_6

24–72 h, the rate was 7.2%; and with a PROM time >72 h, the rate was 9.6%. The differences in the positive blood culture rate among different PROM durations were not statistically significant ($\chi^2 = 2.70, p = 0.259$). When examining the pathogenic bacteria involved in neonatal infections caused by PROM, the proportion of G+ bacteria was significantly greater than that of G− bacilli. Bacteria such as *Staphylococcus epidermidis*, human *Staphylococcus*, *Klebsiella pneumoniae*, *Escherichia coli*, and *Staphylococcus haemolyticus* were among the most common strains that induced a neonate infection after PROM and together accounted for more than 75.0% of the positive blood culture results. Fungi are common pathogenic microorganisms that cause premature infant infection after PROM. (3) Excessive obstetric operations: excessive obstetric operations are prone to cause neonatal infections, and bacteria can infect the fetus either directly or through blood circulation.

2. Intrapartum delivery: Intrapartum infection pathogens primarily include G-bacilli (*Escherichia coli*, *Bacillus proteus*, and *Bacillus gasoformans*), *Salmonella*, and group B β-hemolytic streptococcus. (1) Prolonged second stage of labor: a premature rupture of membranes has not yet occurred, but the patients are in a state of extreme tension; the fetal membrane permeability increases, creating favorable conditions for the invasion of pathogens. (2) Precipitate labor: in precipitate labor, it is often difficult to completely disinfect the sites, thus increasing the chances of infection.
3. Postpartum infection: Postpartum infection is the primary cause of late advanced neonatal pneumonia, and the involved pathogens include *Pseudomonas aeruginosa*, *Klebsiella pneumoniae*, and some conditional pathogenic bacteria with low virulence, such as *Staphylococcus*. (1) Close contact with a respiratory tract infection: if infants inhale air that contains pathogenic microorganisms, various viruses and bacteria can lead to infection after birth. (2) Spread through blood: in cases of damage, infection, and sepsis of the skin and mucous membranes in newborns, pathogens can spread to the lungs through blood circulation. (3) Iatrogenic infection: pathogen accumulation is induced by excessive invasive operations, careless device disinfection, non-strict implementation of sterile operations for working personnel, damage to the integrity of infantile skin during puncture and care, or a drafty atmosphere in the nursery or hospital ward.

6.1.2 Pathophysiology

When lesions are primarily located in the alveoli, alveolar wall congestion, edema, inflammatory cell infiltration, and exudate filling, the alveoli are pathologically visible, causing a reduction in the alveolar diffusion area, an increase in the thickness of the blood gas barrier film, an extension of the diffusion time, and a reduction of the diffusing capacity. During the early stage, alveolar lesions are primarily influenced by the diffusion of oxygen, while during the late stage, they are caused by CO_2 retention. Because the oxygen diffusion capacity decreases, some of the venous blood is transported to the pulmonary veins and the arterial system without being oxygenated in the lungs, leading to a reduction of the arterial partial pressure of oxygen and an increase in the alveolar-arterial oxygen tension difference (A-aDO_2). During severe pneumonia, due to severe hypoxia, pulmonary vascular endothelial cells become swollen, pulmonary vessels become spasmodic and paralytic, pulmonary artery pressure increases, pulmonary capillary permeability increases, blood oozing and flow are slowed, and the lung ventilation/perfusion ratio imbalance worsens, leading to progressive hypoxia and, in severe cases, pulmonary bleeding.

When the lesions are primarily located in the bronchioles and capillary bronchi, the respiratory tract wall is edematous, with inflammatory exudation and increased secretions, causing bronchiolar spasms and ventilation disorders. When the airway is not completely blocked, the inspiration of air is greater than the expiration of air, causing emphysema, decreased alveolar ventilation, and a decreased ventilation/perfusion ratio.

When the airway is completely blocked, some alveoli collapse, atelectasis occurs, the alveolar ventilation/perfusion ratio decreases and becomes further aggravated, and hypoxia is more obvious.

Hypoxia can indirectly stimulate intra-alveolar stretch receptors, which can partially compensate for hypoxia through reflections, tachypnea, and increasing the ventilatory capacity increase, but in cases of serious lung disease or obviously obstructed airways, the compensatory effect is poor and compensation fails. The oxygen consumption of respiratory muscles accounts for 3–5% of the systemic muscle consumption under normal circumstances; in cases where hypoxia cannot be relieved, the infants experience labored respiration, and accessory respiratory muscles are used, causing the oxygen consumption to increase to 5–10 times the normal level, and respiratory failure can be induced due to respiratory muscle fatigue.

6.1.3 Pathology

In cases of intrauterine infectious pneumonia, no special mechanisms are observed. When examined under a microscope, alveoli are involved and full of polynuclear neutrophils and monocytes, erythrocytes are occasionally observed, and the rare exudation of fibrin occurs. Some alveoli have ectasia and contain contents, such as amniotic fluid. In cases of pneumonia caused by the infection of the intrauterine blood circulatory system, alveoli do not contain amniotic fluid contents, but there is a relatively large amount of fibrin exudation.

6.1.4 Clinical Manifestations

1. Intrauterine infectious pneumonia: The onset of intrauterine infectious pneumonia is often early and primarily occurs within 3 days following birth; the patients often have a medical history of asphyxia, and severe intrauterine infections can cause intrauterine fetal death. The manifestations include no crying at birth, difficulty breathing after resuscitation, and the presence of three depression signs, including moaning, cyanosis, and foaming at the mouth. Cough is rare and apnea can be observed. Temperature does not rise or is normal, lung auscultation may indicate that no obvious abnormality is observed, and, sometimes, the symptoms and signs are absent. The primary manifestations of ascending infection are respiratory system symptoms, such as faster breathing, moaning, and abnormal body temperature; in severe cases, the patient can experience respiratory failure, heart failure, convulsions, coma, DIC, shock, and persistent pulmonary hypertension, and lung auscultation indicates that rales and rhonchi can be heard. Hematogenous infections are primarily manifested as jaundice, hepatosplenomegaly, retinal choroiditis, meningoencephalitis, and other multi-system syndromes (fetal lungs are in a compressed state, with the majority of the pulmonary blood flow entering the aorta through the artery catheter and only a small part being diverted into the lungs), and the primary manifestation in the lungs is interstitial pneumonia, usually without rales. Cord blood IgM measurements are >200–300 mg/L, and the specific IgM increase indicates the diagnostic value. The manifestation observed in a chest X-ray examination of those with bacterial infection is usually bronchial pneumonia, while, in those with viral infections, the primary manifestation is interstitial pneumonia.
2. Infectious pneumonia during delivery: Infection is caused by common pathogens (the most common is *E. coli*, followed by *Streptococcus pneumoniae*, *Klebsiella*, *Listeria*, and group B hemolytic streptococci), *Chlamydia trachomatis*, herpes simplex virus, and mycoplasma. The time of onset and the type of infection pathogen are related, and the onset is generally late, appearing after a certain incubation stage. *Chlamydia trachomatis* infection often occurs after 5–14 days, with manifestations of purulent conjunctivitis and the presence of inclusion bodies in conjunctival epithelial cells, and *Chlamydia trachomatis* can be isolated from the nasopharynx. A

cough, which is paroxysmal, without heat or fever, occurs only after 2–12 weeks, and fine crackles can be observed in the lungs; the manifestation observed in the chest X-ray is local interstitial pneumonia. During herpes simplex virus infection, herpes can be observed on the head skin at birth, appearing 5–10 days after birth, and the symptom of meningitis is often more prominent. Bacteria (such as *E. coli* and other intestinal bacteria)-induced pneumonia usually occurs 3–10 days after birth; in addition to respiratory symptoms, it often leads to sepsis, and the onset occurs as an even outbreak with a high mortality; chest X-ray examinations present the manifestation of bronchopneumonia.

3. Infectious pneumonia after birth: The routes of pathogen invasion include descending infection (pathogens spread through droplets from the respiratory tract to the lungs), hematogenous infection, and iatrogenic infections (such as ventilator-associated pneumonia, the use of broad-spectrum antibiotics). A variety of viruses, bacteria, and other microorganisms can cause pneumonia infection after birth, and the common pathogens of ventilator-associated pneumonia are *Klebsiella pneumoniae*, *Pseudomonas aeruginosa*, and *Escherichia coli*. Those who undergo the long-term use of broad-spectrum antibiotics are prone to experience *Candida albicans* pneumonia, and those with immune deficiencies are susceptible to *Pneumocystis carinii* pneumonitis. The respiratory symptoms include difficulty breathing, flaring of nares, spittle, cyanosis, nodding breathing, and restractions, but pulmonary symptoms are not typical. Respiratory syncytial virus pneumonia may be manifested as wheezing, and lung auscultation indicates that wheeze can be heard. Pneumonia caused by different pathogens may have different results from chest X-ray examinations, with the primary manifestation of viral infection being interstitial pneumonia and the primary manifestation of bacterial infection being bronchial pneumonia. *Staphylococcus aureus* infections are apt to be complicated by empyema and pyopneumothorax. Bacterial culture of nasopharyngeal secretions, virus isolation, fluorescent antibody tests, and serum-specific antibody tests is used to aid in the etiological diagnosis.
4. Common Complications
   (a) Congestive heart failure: In cases of pneumonia, heart failure often occurs due to the following reasons:
      - Hypoxic acidosis induces pulmonary vascular spasms and increased pulmonary artery pressure.
      - Inflammatory exudation causes pulmonary edema, increasing the before and afterload and causing right heart failure.
      - Myocardial hypoxia-ischemia, energy metabolism disorder, bacterial toxins, acidosis, and electrolyte imbalance induce the cardiac muscle cell to experience ultrastructural damage, excitation-contraction coupling disorder, and decreased myocardial contractility.
      - Lower diastolic blood pressure and decreased coronary blood flow may further weaken myocardial contractility.
      - In cases of severe pneumonia, under the influence of bacterial toxins, the peripheral α-receptor is excited, vasoconstriction occurs, and the left heart afterload increases, causing a decrease in cardiac output; simultaneously, the sympathetic nerve excitation causes the redistribution of systemic blood flow, decreases the renal blood flow, activates the renin-angiotensin-aldosterone system, causes an increase in water and sodium retention and the returned blood volume, and increases cardiac preload, causing congestive heart failure.

   (b) Acid-base balance disorder: In cases of severe pneumonia, due to an increase in anaerobic metabolism, a large amount of lactic acid is generated, causing lactic acidosis and leading to metabolic acidosis. During the early stages, hypoxia may be complicated by mild respiratory alkalosis, due to ventilatory compensation; the seriousness and progression of patient conditions cause CO_2 retention and induce mixed acidosis. However, metabolic alkalosis rarely occurs except in the case of excessive alkali supplementation or improper mechanical ventilation during the treatment. When the pH <7.2, kidney function becomes involved, urination is stopped, liver function is impaired, and the activity of enzymes involved in the metabolism of bilirubin is inhibited, which can induce bilirubin encephalopathy; during acidosis, the response of the body to catecholamines weakens and dysemia occurs. When the pH <7.0, myocardial glucose metabolism is fully terminated, followed by circulatory failure and cerebral hypoxic injuries.

(c) Water and electrolyte balance disorder: In cases of pneumonia, fever and tachypnea increase the loss of water and electrolytes from the respiratory tract and the skin, and hypertonic dehydration may occur; if accompanied by vomiting and diarrhea, which can further exacerbate the loss of water from the body, dehydration can become further aggravated.

Potassium metabolism disorders: The following factors often cause elevated serum potassium levels in infants: (1) in cases of acidosis, the H^+ concentration in plasma increases, and H^+ enters into cells, through the H^+/K^+ exchange, causing K^+ to be released from cells and inducing intercellular fluid; and (2) in cases of infection, cell injury, glycogen, and protein decomposition induce K^+ release, leading to the elevation of serum potassium levels. However, the total in vivo potassium decreases in infants for the following reasons: (a) renal compensation causes an increase in K^+ excretion; in cases of dehydration, reflexivity increases the secretion of aldosterone, causing an increase in the renal excretion of K^+; (b) inadequate K^+ intake; (c) loss due to vomiting and diarrhea; and (d) the neonatal ability to secrete antidiuretic hormones is immature and renal K^+ retention is relatively weak.

In cases of metabolic acidosis, the plasma HCO_3^- content decreases; in addition to lactic acidosis, the plasma Cl^- level also increases with the occurrence of hyperchloremic acidosis. In cases of respiratory acidosis, the blood $H_2CO_3^-$ concentration significantly increases and the renal compensatory reabsorption of $H_2CO_3^-$ and the discharge of Cl^- increase, causing hypochloremic acidosis.

(d) Cerebral edema and toxic encephalopathy: Cerebral edema is relatively common in patients with ventilatory disorders. Because CO_2 retention and acidosis induce cephalemia and telangiectasia, blood capillaries become dilated, the vascular permeability increases with exoserosis, and local microcirculatory disturbances occur in the brain to produce intercellular edema (angioedema). Hypoxia, acidosis, and low blood sugar induce energy metabolism disorders, decreasing the activity of the $Na^+/K^+/$ ATPase, causing Na^+ and H_2O to enter the cells but making them difficult to be discharged from the cells, and resulting in edema. In addition, electrolyte imbalances and sodium retention further exacerbate cerebral edema. Severe cerebral edema can induce an increase in intracranial pressure, often accompanied by convulsions and even leading to brain herniation.

(e) Toxic enteroparalysis: Severe pneumonia increases catecholamine secretion; redistributes blood flow; induces gastrointestinal tract microcirculation disorders, intestinal ischemia, passive hyperemia of the lungs, hypoxia, edema, and exudation; reduces intestinal motility and smooth muscle relaxation; and induces intestinal paralysis and aeration. Hypokalemia can cause enteroparalysis. Serious intestinal gas causes the diaphragmatic muscles to increase, limiting lung ventilation and further aggravating infant dyspnea.

(f) Renal impairment: Due to the total redistribution of blood flow, renal blood flow is also reduced; a reduced glomerular filtration rate may cause sodium retention. Long-term ischemia and hypoxia can lead to tubular necrosis and renal failure.
(g) Pulmonary hemorrhage: In cases of acidosis, blood viscosity increases, causing slowed blood flow, and late infectious pneumonia is often complicated by polycythemia and a reduced tendency toward deformation, which causes embolization; shock also can cause blood stasis and thrombosis. The deposition of IgG, C3, and antigen-antibody complexes on capillary basement membranes can induce pulmonary vascular injury and blood leakage; congestive cardiac failure increases pulmonary vascular pressure and resistance, inducing pulmonary edema, and the occurrence of pulmonary hemorrhage can be promoted.
(h) Hypoglycemia: In cases of serious infections, glucose consumption triples, and the activity of the enzyme that promotes gluconeogenesis in the neonate liver is relatively low, so that it is not difficult to transform amino acids into glucose. In cases of aggravated infections, the brown fat becomes exhausted, and gluconeogenesis is reduced so that hypoglycemia is apt to occur. In addition, fever and increased respiratory movement both increase sugar consumption, and low food intake, vomiting, and gastrointestinal dysfunction decrease the intake of exogenous sources of energy, which can cause or aggravate the occurrence of hypoglycemia.
(i) Circulatory disorder and shock: In cases of severe pneumonia, anoxia, toxins, acidosis, heart failure, stress, and other reasons can cause microcirculation disorders, resulting in small blood vascular spasms and reduced blood supply, and the opening of capillaries causes microcirculatory blood flow stasis, inducing shock, disseminated intravascular coagulation, and organ necrosis.
(j) Disseminated intravascular coagulation (DIC): The effects of hypoxia and endotoxins induce vascular endothelial injuries, acidosis induces vasodilation and slow blood flow, and shock induces microcirculation stasis and plasma exosmosis, causing and aggravating ischemic hypoxia, anoxia, and acidosis and initiating the endogenous coagulation pathway that leads to DIC. In addition, during the neonatal period, the plasma clotting factor content is low, the content of hemoglobin is high, and blood viscosity is high, and the ability of the liver to synthesize clotting factors is low, making DIC apt to occur to neonates. The combined effects of the above factors increase the likelihood of neonates to experience DIC in cases of serious pneumonia.

6.1.5 Auxiliary Examination

1. Conventional examinations: Routine blood test, CRP, and blood culture.
2. Chest X-ray examination: (1) For pneumonia induced by intrauterine and delivery processes, no abnormal findings can be found during X-ray examination on the first day after birth, and the following changes can occur 24 h thereafter: changes of interstitial pneumonia; the lungs become full of small, patchy or linear, blurred shadows, which become a diffuse fan shape around the pulmonary portae; the bronchial walls become thickened; and particle-shaped shadows are observed, accompanied by air bronchogram and emphysema. (2) Pneumonia after birth often has the following manifestations: a wide range of spot-shaped and patch infiltration shadows in the lung field, likely accompanied by emphysema and atelectasis; occasional large lobar consolidation with empyema, pyopneumothorax, lung abscess, and bunamiodyl; diffuse blurred shadows in both lungs, varying in shadow density and depth, with bacterial pneumonia being common; and cord-shaped shadows in two pulmonary por-

tae and interstitia of lung fields, likely accompanied by scattered pulmonary infiltration and obvious emphysema, with virus pneumonia being common.

6.1.6 Treatment

1. Strengthen nursing, maintain body temperature and maintain a neutral ambient temperature, and prevent disease progression and deterioration.
2. Strengthen respiratory tract management: Receive physical therapies, such as aerosol inhalation, postural drainage, and regular turning-over and back-tapping, and maintain smooth airway.
3. Oxygen supply: Maintain the arterial blood PaO_2 concentration at 50–80 mmHg. Hoods can be used for oxygen supply; in severe cases, CPAP and even breathing machines may be used for treatment. Attention should be paid to the following problems when using oxygen therapy: (1) If the diseases are accompanied by severe hypoxemia induced by CO_2 retention, high concentrations of oxygen should be given; because CO_2 paralysis cannot excite the respiratory center, suppression of peripheral chemoreceptors cannot stimulate the respiratory center and can inhibit spontaneous respiration. (2) Measures should be adopted to gradually reduce oxygen concentration after hypoxemia symptoms have improved following oxygen therapy; otherwise, the oxygen concentration will plunge, inducing sudden pulmonary spasms and leading to pulmonary hypertension and right to left shunt, which is difficult to reverse.
4. Pathogenetic therapy: Bacterial pneumonia should be treated intravenously with antibiotics; however, it is often difficult to quickly determine the responsible pathogen. Cephalosporins can be administered, and the categories of antibiotics used can be adjusted according to the patient's conditions. Penicillin can be given to treat group B β-hemolytic streptococcus, ampicillin can be given to treat *Listeria* pneumonia, erythromycin can be given to treat chlamydia and mycoplasma, acyclovir can be used to treat herpes simplex virus, ganciclovir can be used to treat cytomegalovirus pneumonia, and 200,000–1,000,000 U/day of intramuscularly injected α1-interference is effective against viral pneumonia, with the treatment courses ranging from 5 to 7 days.
5. Support therapy: Circulation disorder and water-electrolyte disorder should be corrected, with a daily total liquid volume of 60–80 ml/kg and a slow infusion speed to avoid pulmonary edema and heart failure and ensure adequate calories. Albumin and immunoglobulin infusion can be given as needed to improve the body immune function.

6.2 Ultrasound Diagnosis of Infectious Pneumonia

Lung ultrasound has been increasingly used for the diagnosis and differential diagnosis of severe lung disease in the field of critical care medicine, and it is rarely used in the diagnosis of neonatal pneumonia, which is not domestically reported. Based on the experience of using ultrasound for the diagnosis of infectious pneumonia in infants and adults, we investigated the value of applying ultrasound to the diagnosis of infectious pneumonia in neonatal lungs (the study protocol was approved by the institutional review board of the Beijing Military General Hospital and Beijing Chaoyang District Maternal and Child Health Care Hospital), and the results confirmed that using real-time ultrasound for the diagnosis of neonatal infectious pneumonia was accurate and reliable, with a relatively high sensitivity and specificity. The primary ultrasound imaging features of neonate infectious pneumonia include a massive area of pulmonary consolidation with air bronchogram, abnormalities of pleural lines, AIS or pulmonary edema, and the disappearance of A-lines [4–7].

Lung consolidation with air bronchogram is the primary basis for using ultrasound to diagnose pneumonia, which is characterized by [5–8]:

1. Hypoechoic areas with varying size and shape (irregular consolidation area), and usually a

larger consolidation range, with irregular borders and a jagged shape.

2. Consolidation with irregular jagged edges with air bronchogram. The consolidation can be located in any part of the lung field.
3. In cases of serious and large-scale consolidation, using real-time ultrasound, the air movement in the bronchi can be observed, which is known as dynamic air bronchogram.
4. Color Doppler ultrasound can indicate the pulmonary blood flow signals in the consolidation area. Color or energy Doppler can indicate the pulmonary blood flow signals in the consolidation area, showing that blood supply is present in the consolidated lung tissues, which is necessary for pulmonary lesions to recover or heal.
5. Pleural effusion may be present to varying degrees. It can be differentiated with RDS and MAS, according to the above features.

Neonatal infectious pneumonia is common, and nonspecific ultrasound changes include abnormalities in pleural line ultrasound abnormalities, the disappearance of the A-line and AIS. Abnormal pleural lines and AIS are related to inflammatory exudation, and, in severe cases, a small amount of pleural effusion can be noted. Because A-line is the reflection line of the pleural line, abnormalities of pleural line must be accompanied by abnormal A-lines, which is primarily manifested as the disappearance of the A-line. The above symptoms are also observed in other lung diseases, such as RDS, MAS, and TTN, and are not specific to IPN [8].

The disappearance of lung sliding and lung pulse under real-time ultrasound are important imaging features of neonatal infectious pneumonia, and we observed that 84.4% of newborns with infectious pneumonia showed varying degrees of lung pulse and the disappearance of lung side when examined using real-time ultrasound. Lung pulse is also found in severe atelectasis, suggesting that the existence and extent of lung pulse are associated with the formation and extent of pulmonary consolidation and/or atelectasis, and it is considered to be one of the characteristic symptoms of atelectasis.

Lung consolidation is the necessary ultrasonographic observation for the diagnosis of pulmonary atelectasis and RDS. However, in the case of atelectasis, the edges of pulmonary consolidation areas are relatively clear and regular, and usually one site of consolidation is observed in one lateral field and often in an air bronchogram that is arranged in parallel; in pneumonia, multiple consolidations can be observed, and a dynamic air bronchogram is common. The consolidation of RDS begins from the subpleural regions and is associated with the range and extent of the lesion, and the air bronchogram in consolidation areas presents a relatively fine, short, linear shape. Of course, a truly accurate identification not only requires adequate knowledge and experience using a lung ultrasound but also the combination of the medical history and clinical manifestations, which is the advantage of a neonatal physician performing the ultrasound examination.

Please see the related pictures and movie in Figs. 6.1–6.16 and Video 6.1.

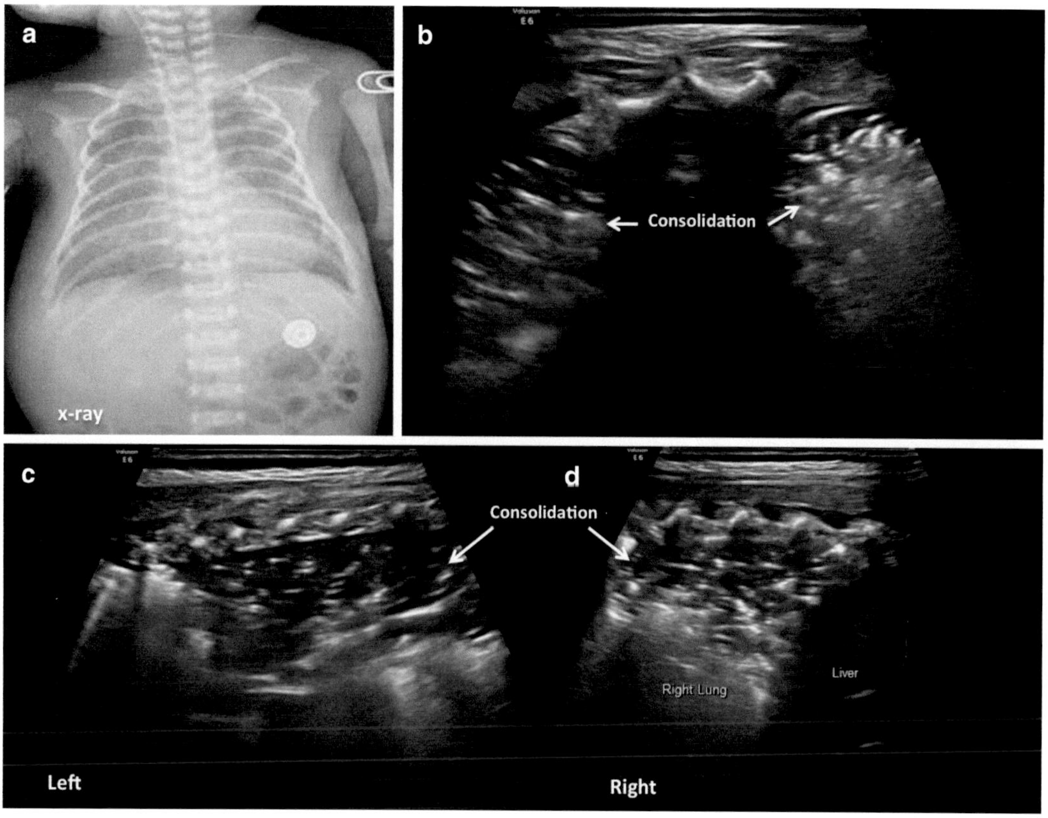

Fig. 6.1 Ultrasound manifestations of infectious pneumonia. Gestational age of 38^{+2} weeks, delivered by cesarean section, with a birth weight of 3420 g. The patient was admitted due to dyspnea 3 days after birth. Temperature was 38 °C, and dense moist rales were heard in both lungs. Routine blood test results: WBC 22×10^9/L, N% 78%, MONO% 12.2%, and CRP 66.8 mg/L. Chest X-ray (**a**) shows significant pneumonia in bilateral lungs. Lung ultrasound shows large-scale consolidation areas with irregular margins and air bronchogram; part of the pleural line disappears, and the remaining parts present changes consistent with alveolar interstitial syndrome, with the disappearance of A-lines (**c**, **d**). The infant is lying in the prone position and is scanned through the transverse section of the spinal column, and the results further display the presence of consolidation in both lungs (**b**)

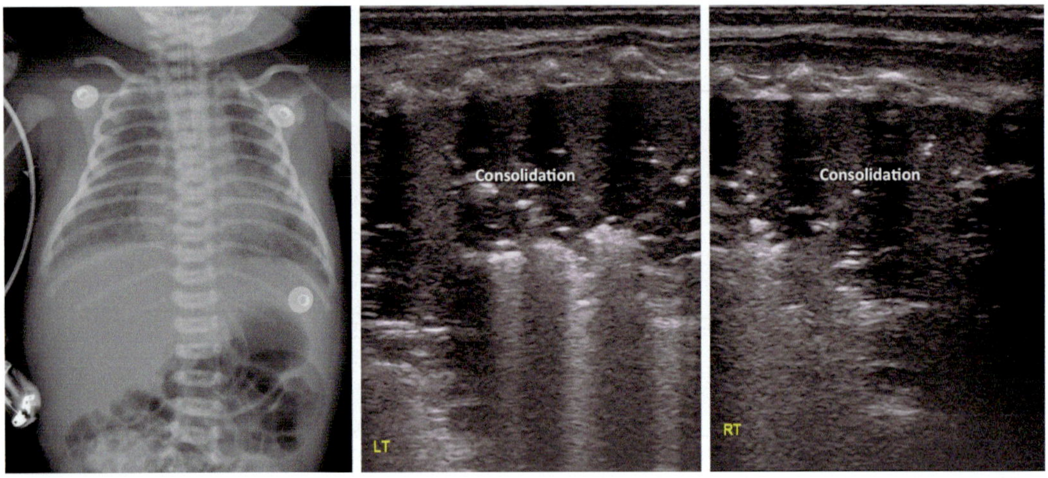

Fig. 6.2 Ultrasound manifestations of infectious pneumonia. Gestational age of 37 weeks, delivered by cesarean section, with a birth weight of 3700 g. No asphyxia, history of PROM, dyspnea after birth, or fever. Routine blood test results: WBC 30 × 10^9/L, N% 81% mononuclear PLT 67 × 10^9/L, CRP 39 mg/L. Lung ultrasound reveals a large area of consolidation with irregular edges, accompanied by air bronchogram in bilateral lung fields; the pleural line is present; the A-line disappears. The chest X-ray indicates neonatal pneumonia with obvious manifestations in both sides of the lungs

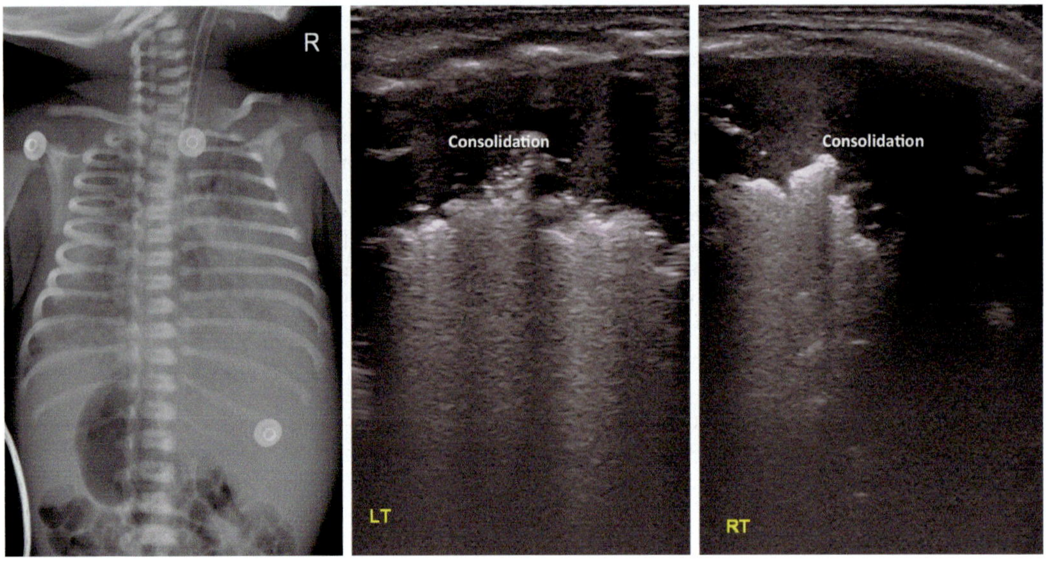

Fig. 6.3 Ultrasound manifestations of infectious pneumonia. Gestational age of 38 weeks and a birth weight of 4200 g. The patient was admitted for 3 days due to dyspnea with fever, and dense moist rales were heard in the lungs. In combination with a routine blood test and chest X-ray examinations, the diagnosis was severe pneumonia in both sides of the lungs. Lung ultrasound reveals a large area of consolidation with irregular edges and uneven internal echoes in the bilateral lung fields, accompanied by air bronchogram (left lung, the probe is perpendicular to the ribs; right lung, the probe is parallel to the ribs)

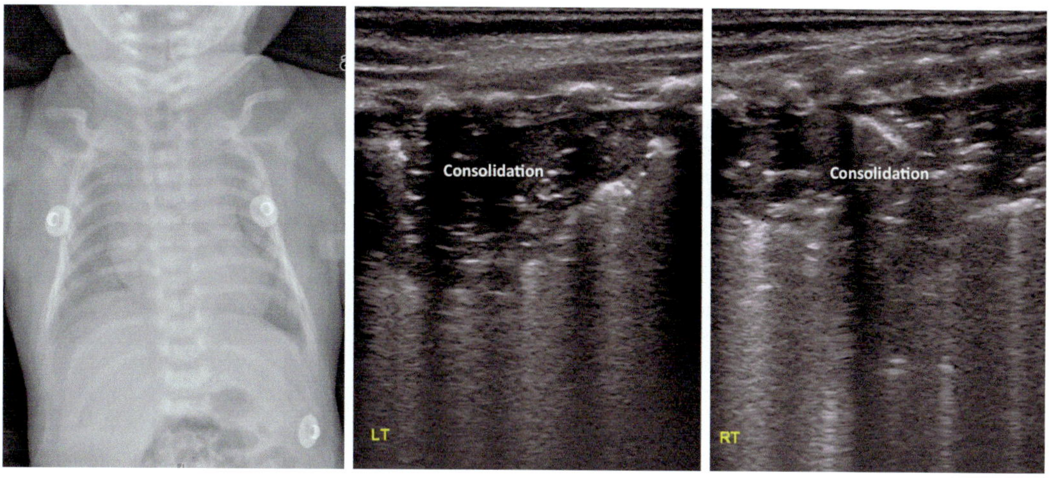

Fig. 6.4 Ultrasound manifestations of infectious pneumonia. Gestational age of 35^{+1} weeks, spontaneous labor, and a birth weight of 1850 g. PROM occurred 49 h prior to the examination, and the amniotic fluid was turbid. Not long after birth, the patient experienced dyspnea with a low temperature and received respiratory treatment. Routine blood test results: WBC 2980 × 10^9/L, N87%, PLT 87 × 10^9/L, and blood culture indicated the growth of *Klebsiella pneumoniae*. Chest X-ray shows a shadow with increased density in the right lung, with obvious manifestations at the right lower lung. Lung ultrasound reveals large areas of consolidation in the bilateral lung fields, accompanied by significant air bronchogram; the pleural line partially disappears, and the A-line disappears

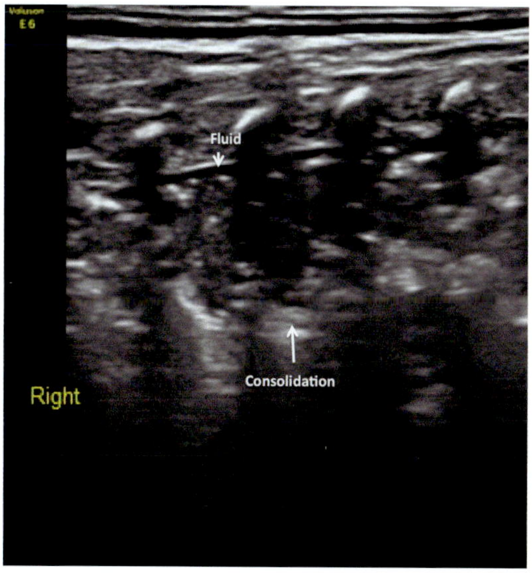

Fig. 6.5 Ultrasound manifestations of infectious pneumonia. Gestational age of 37 weeks and a birth weight of 2150 g. The patient was admitted due to fever and breathing difficulties 2 days after birth, and lung auscultation indicated dense rales. A significant elevation was observed in the WBC, N%, and CRP, as indicated in the routine blood test results, and the chest X-ray is consistent with the changes observed in pneumonia. Lung ultrasound shows large consolidation shadows with irregular, jagged edges, accompanied by air bronchograms; the A-line disappears, some of the pleural line disappears, and a very small amount of pleural effusion was observed

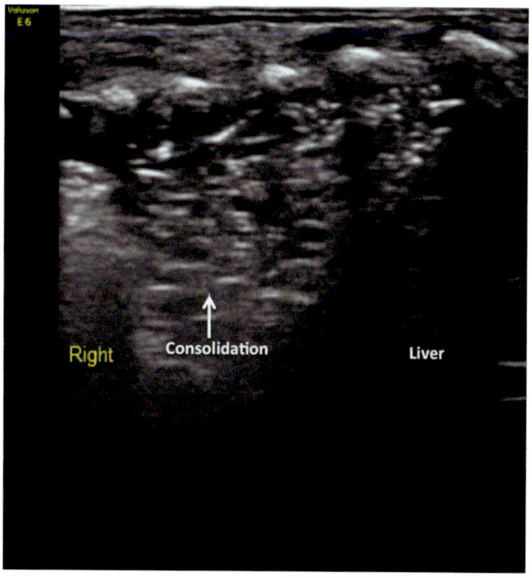

Fig. 6.6 Ultrasound manifestations of infectious pneumonia. This was a premature newborn infant with a gestational age of 30^{+1} weeks, and chest X-ray shows right lower lung pneumonia. The ultrasound shows a large area of consolidation, with significant air bronchograms, in the right lower lung field

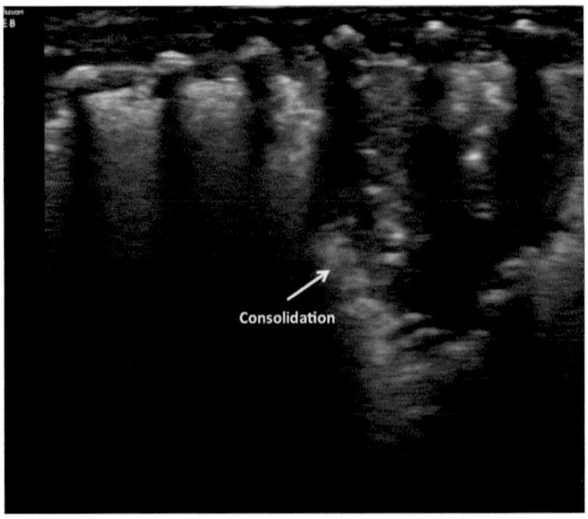

Fig. 6.7 Ultrasound manifestations of infectious pneumonia. Gestational age of 33^{+4} weeks and a birth weight of 1650 g. The patient was admitted for 3 days due to dyspnea with fever and received ventilator treatment. Chest X-ray examination shows double markings that have become thickened, blurred, and disorderly, and visible chunks of dense shadow are observed in right lower lung. In combination with the clinical manifestations, the diagnosis was pneumonia. Lung ultrasound shows three intercostal consolidation shadows in the right lung field, and the margins of the consolidation areas in the deep area of the lung fields present jagged edges, accompanied by air bronchogram; the remaining parts present significant alveolar-interstitial syndrome, with disappearing pleural and A-lines

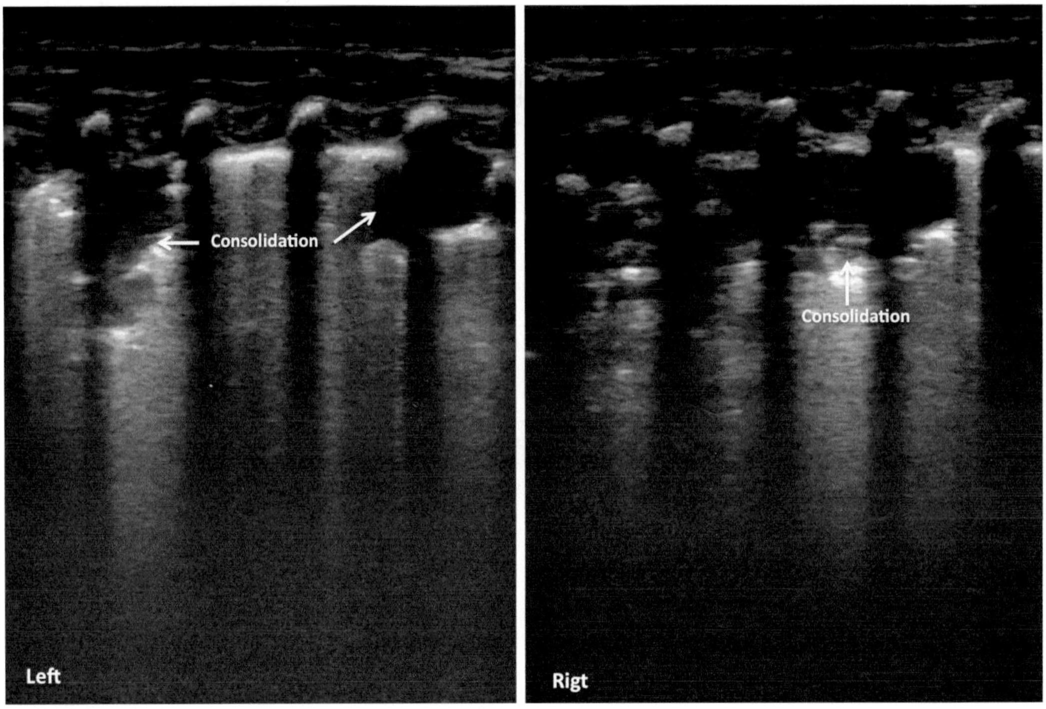

Fig. 6.8 Different areas of lung consolidation in pneumonia. Ultrasound examination shows the presence of different areas of lung consolidation in different regions of lung fields accompanied by an air bronchogram. In combination with clinical manifestations, laboratory tests, and a chest X-ray, the diagnosis is infectious pneumonia. The presence of different degrees and different ranges of consolidation in the lung fields is one of the important ultrasound manifestations of neonate infectious pneumonia, and the heterogeneity of intrapulmonary lesions of pneumonia is reflected

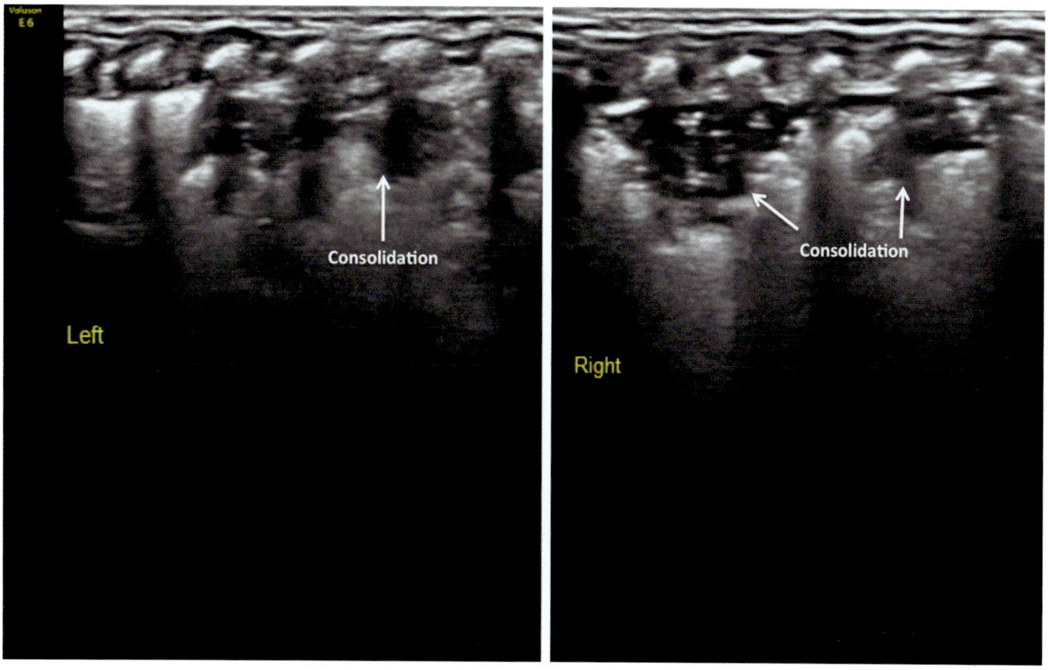

Fig. 6.9 Different areas of lung consolidation in pneumonia. Gestational age of 38^{+5} weeks, delivered by cesarean section, with no asphyxia and a birth weight of 3935 g. The patient experienced dyspnea soon after birth, the body temperature was 39 °C, and a large quantity of moist rales could be heard in the lungs. Routine blood test results: WBC 22 × 10^9/L, N% 89.1%, CRP 31 mg/L. Lung ultrasound reveals a large area of consolidation with irregular edges in the left lung, and different consolidation areas with different sizes and shapes are observed, all accompanied by air bronchogram

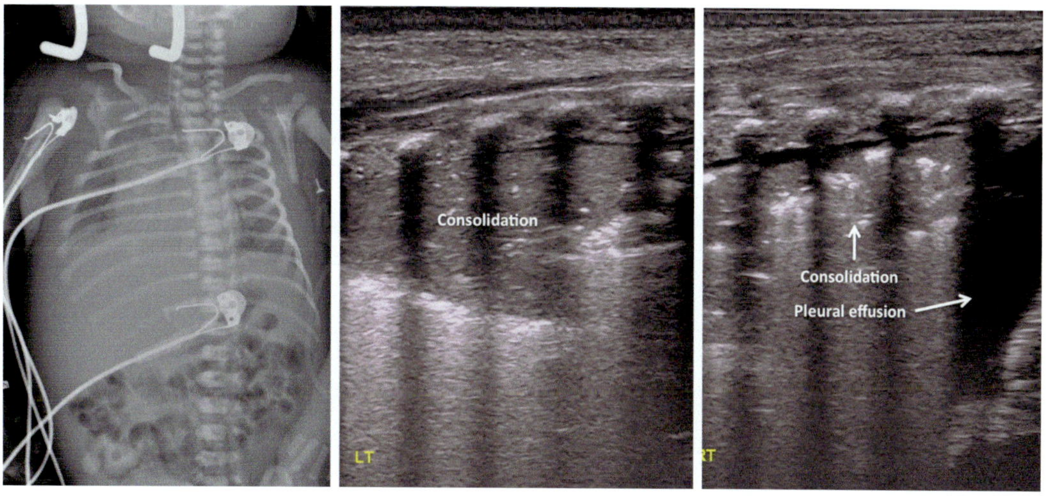

Fig. 6.10 Pleural effusion in pneumonia patient. Gestational age of 38^{+3} weeks and a birth weight of 3270 g. The patient was admitted to the hospital 5 h after birth because of pneumonia, which was diagnosed according to clinical manifestation and chest X-ray findings. Lung ultrasound showed large areas of consolidation with significant air bronchograms in bilateral lung fields, as well as pleural effusion, which is more significant in the right lung

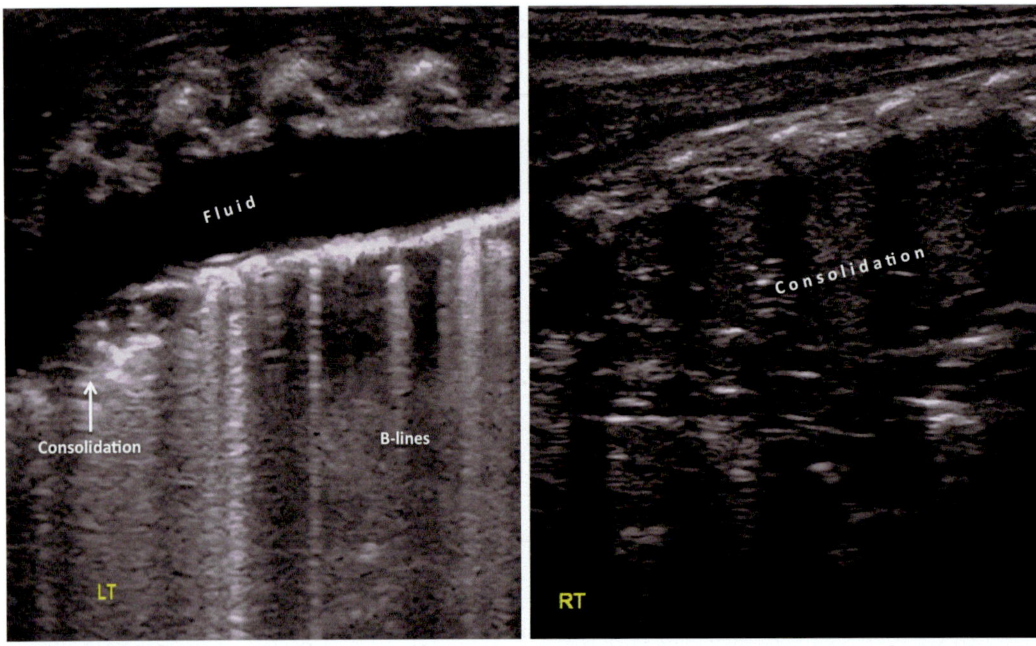

Fig. 6.11 Different ultrasonic findings for different sides of the lungs in a pneumonia patient. Gestational age of 33^{+4} weeks and a birth weight of 1650 g. The patient was admitted for 3 days due to dyspnea with fever and received ventilator treatment. In combination with the clinical manifestations, the diagnosis was pneumonia. Lung ultrasound shows different findings for different sides of the lungs; the left lung primarily manifested as a pleural effusion with a small area of consolidation, with B-lines and disappearing A-lines, and the right lung primarily presented with a large area of consolidation with air bronchograms

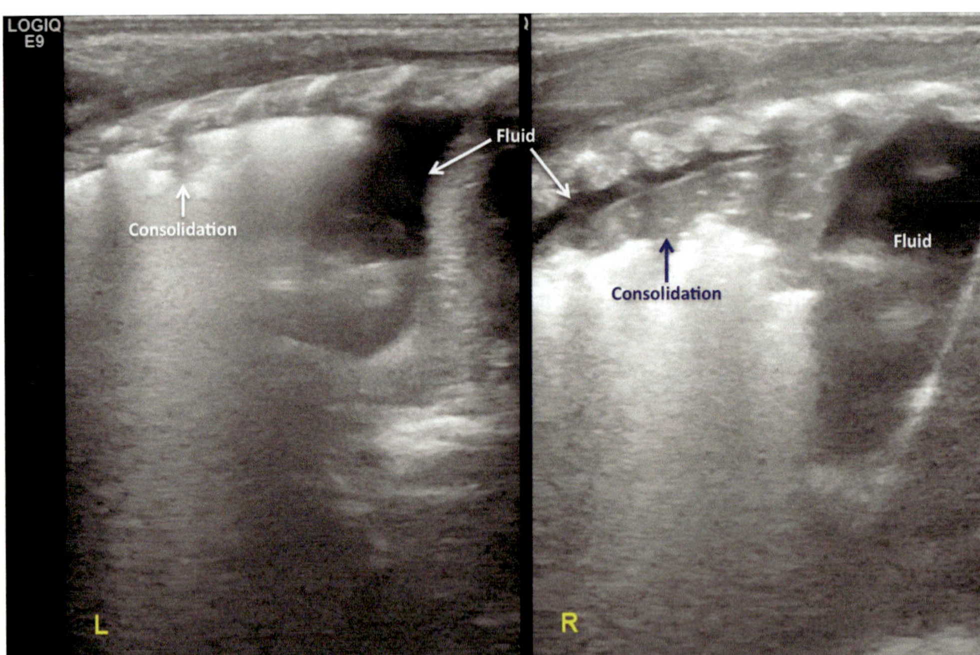

Fig. 6.12 Ultrasound manifestations of infectious pneumonia. This baby was admitted to the NICU because of severe anemia with significant dyspnea. The ultrasound shows significant levels of fluid in the bilateral chest, a large area of consolidation in the right lung and a small consolidation in the left lung, abnormal pleural lines and disappearing A-lines

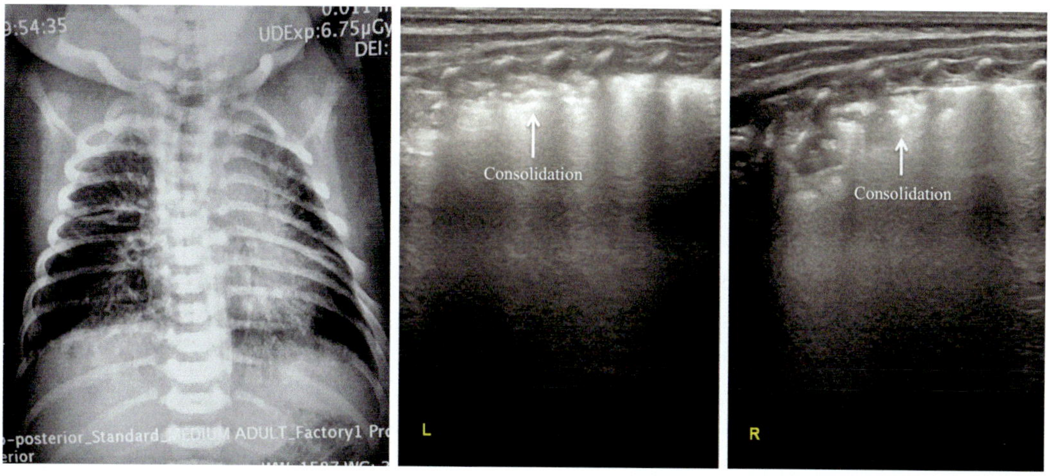

Fig. 6.13 Subpleural consolidation in mild pneumonia. The baby was diagnosed with mild pneumonia, according to the clinical information and chest X-ray manifestation. Ultrasound shows a mild subpleural consolidation in the left lung field and a relatively significant consolidation in the right lung field

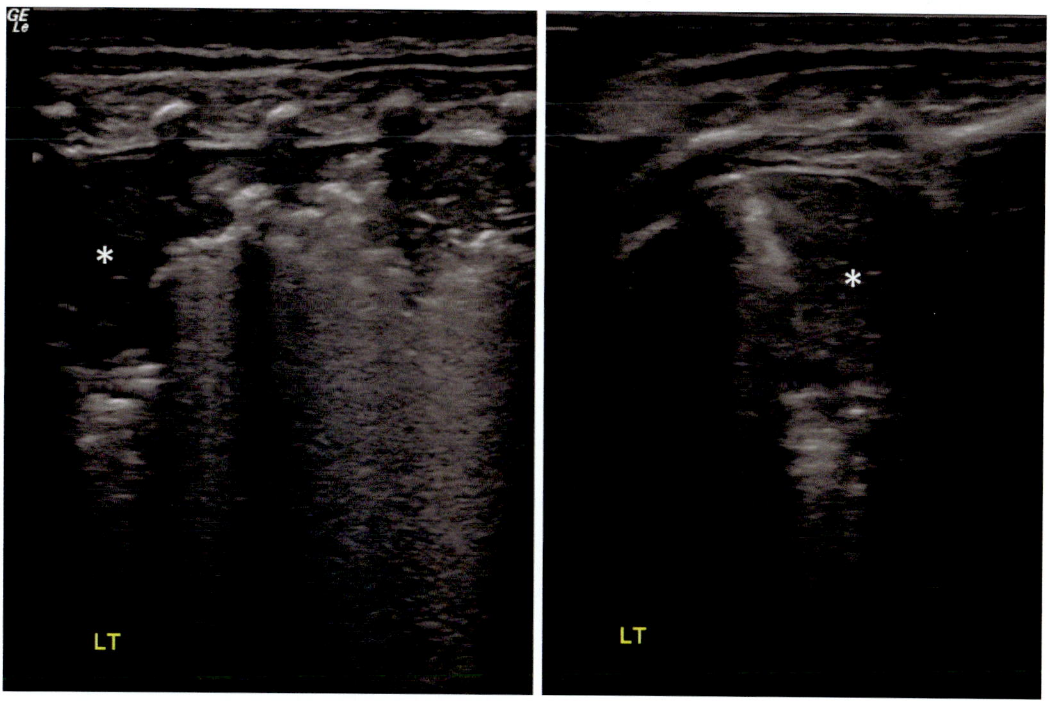

Fig. 6.14 Ventilator-associated pneumonia. A neonatal patient with ventilator-associated pneumonia. Lung ultrasound shows a very large area of lung consolidation, with significant air bronchograms and irregular margins in the left lung (left picture, the probe is perpendicular to the ribs; right picture, the probe is parallel to the ribs)

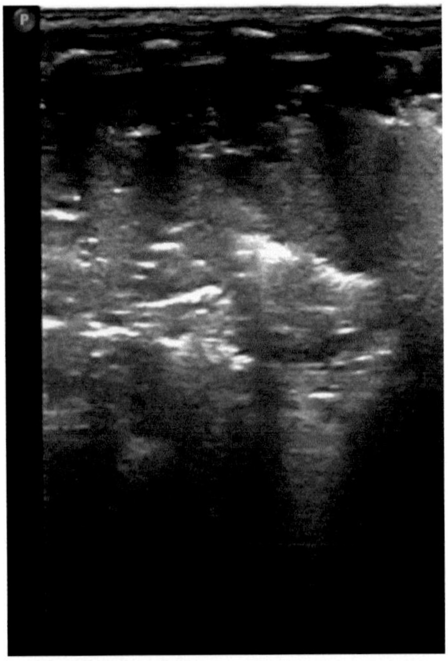

Fig. 6.15 Dynamic air bronchograms in severe pneumonia patients. The ultrasound shows a very large area of consolidation, with significant air bronchograms, in a severe pneumonia patient, and the significant, dynamic air bronchograms can be observed using real-time ultrasound (Video 6.1)

References

1. Guo YM, Liu CQ. The clinical epidemiology of neonatal respiratory failure in Hebei Children's Hospital. Zhonghua Weichan Yixue Zazhi. 2012;15(11):670–5.
2. Rao Y. Analysis of 7970 cases in-hospital newborn infants. Zhongguo Bing An. 2012;13(1):71–3.
3. Zhao H, Jin ZJ. Analysis of death reasons in 1509 newborn infants. Zhongguo Fu You Jian Kang Yan Jiu. 2009;20(5):686–8.
4. Reissig A, Gramegna A, Aliberti S. The role of lung ultrasound in the diagnosis and follow-up of community-acquired pneumonia. Eur J Intern Med. 2012;23(5):391–7.
5. Caiulo VA, Gargani L, Caiulo S, et al. Lung ultrasound characteristics of community-acquired pneumonia in hospitalized children. Pediatr Pulmonol. 2013;48(3):280–7.
6. Cortellaro F, Colombo S, Coen D, et al. Lung ultrasound is an accurate diagnosis too for the diagnosis of pneumonia in the emergency department. Emerg Med J. 2012;29(1):19–23.
7. Raimondi F, Cattarossi L, Copetti R. International perspectives: point-of-care chest ultrasound in the neonatal intensive care unit: an Italian perspective. NeoReviews. 2014;15(1):e2–6.
8. Liu J, Liu F, Liu Y, et al. Lung ultrasonography for the diagnosis of severe pneumonia of the newborn. Chest. 2014;146(2):483–8.

Fig. 6.16 Severe pneumonia (*volume panorama*). A severe pneumonia patient. Lung ultrasound (*volume panorama mode*) showed large area of consolidation involved in the whole left lung, in fact that, atelectasis has already formed in the area of severe consolidated lung tissues.

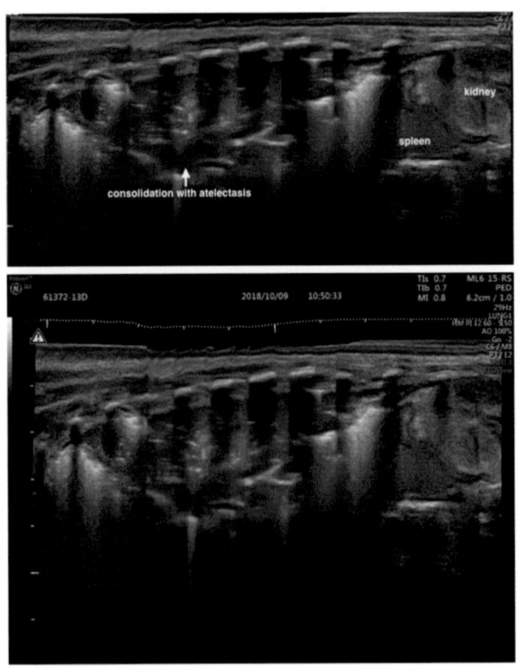

7 Pulmonary Atelectasis of the Newborn

Jing Liu and Hai-Ying Cao

7.1 Pulmonary Atelectasis

In utero, the fetal lungs are atelectatic. Twenty minutes after birth, the lung volume reaches 17 mL, and 3–6 h later, it reaches 36 mL. Full lung dilation usually does not occur for several days. Lung dilation usually starts from the anterior margin and the apex of the lungs, and the paravertebral dilation and central and rear dilation occur later. The inability to undergo pulmonary dilation for any reason, or the loss of normal function in response to inadequate aeration from collapse of the pulmonary tissues, is called atelectasis [1, 2]. Atelectasis is not an independent disease; instead, it is a common complication of multiple diseases. Atelectasis is a common cause of neonatal dyspnea, protracted illness, and difficulty withdrawing a ventilator. The correct diagnosis of atelectasis is important for reasonable treatment, improvement of the patient's condition, and prognosis [1–3].

Electronic Supplementary Material The online version of this chapter (https://doi.org/10.1007/978-94-024-1549-0_7) contains supplementary material, which is available to authorized users.

J. Liu (✉)
Department of Neonatology and NICU,
Beijing Chaoyang District Maternal and Child Health Care Hospital, Beijing, China

H.-Y. Cao
Department of Ultrasound, GE Healthcare,
Beijing, China

7.1.1 Etiology and Pathophysiology [1, 3]

Although many factors can cause neonatal atelectasis, its exact cause is unclear. Neonatal pulmonary atelectasis is more common in premature infants than in-term infants. For example, among the 23 cases of neonatal atelectasis reported by Owens et al., premature infants accounted for 82.6%.

1. Congenital atelectasis: Induced by bronchial congenital dysplasia or aplasia.
2. External compression: For the lung parenchyma or bronchial compression, multiple scenarios are observed, which are summarized here. (1) Thoracic movement disorders: observed in nerve, muscular, and skeletal abnormalities, such as severe central nervous system damage, multiple neurodocitis, spinal muscular atrophy, grave myasthenia, and skeletal deformity. (2) Diaphragmatic movement disorder: observed as diaphragmatic paralysis or significantly increased intra-abdominal cavity pressure. (3) Limited lung dilation: observed with a decrease in the negative intrathoracic pressure or an increase in pressure, such as from significant pleural effusion, pneumatosis, diaphragmatic hernia, tumor, or significantly increased heart size. (4) Bronchi subjected to external pressure: observed with luminal blockage that induces bronchial compression, such that air cannot enter lung

J. Liu et al. (eds.), *Neonatal Lung Ultrasonography*, https://doi.org/10.1007/978-94-024-1549-0_7

tissues. For example, the dilated left atria and pulmonary arteries can compress the left main bronchus, inducing left atelectasis.

3. Obstruction within the bronchi or bronchioles. (1) Foreign body: a foreign body obstructs the bronchi or bronchioles, inducing lobar or segmental pulmonary atelectasis. Larger foreign bodies obstruct organs or main bronchi, inducing bilateral or unilateral atelectasis. (2) Bronchial lesions: tracheal-bronchial softening, airway constriction or dilation, etc. (3) Viscous secretions block the bronchi: in the case of neonatal respiratory tract narrowing, the bronchi can be blocked by viscous secretion, which is the most common reason for neonatal atelectasis. Viscous secretions are seen in pneumonia, meconium aspiration syndrome, respiratory distress syndrome, chronic pulmonary disease, following esophageal atresia repair, etc. Due to bronchial mucosal swelling and smooth muscle spasm, the viscous secretions block the airway, inducing atelectasis.
4. Nonobstructive atelectasis: (1) This case is mainly seen in infants with primary or secondary deficiency of pulmonary surfactants. The surface tension of normal alveoli is 6 dyn/cm^2; however, in the absence of pulmonary surfactant, the lung surface tension of infants with respiratory distress syndrome can be up to 236 dyn/cm^2. The increase in surface tension and increase in the alveolar retractive force cause alveolar collapse, resulting in multiple sites with microatelectasis. (2) Hypopnea can occur in infants with long-term use of sedatives and anesthetics (or even short-term use of high levels), in a coma, or who are extremely weak; when the pressure is insufficient to resist local pulmonary surface tension, it can gradually lead to alveolar closure and anesthesia. Therefore, encouraging or stimulating infants to take a deep breath helps prevent alveolar closure or helps recruit alveoli that would otherwise close with shallow breathing.

7.1.2 Clinical Manifestations [1–5]

1. Unilateral or bilateral atelectasis: The main manifestations are progressive aggravation of dyspnea and cyanosis. Aggravation often occurs after crying or exertion. In the absence of bruising and dyspnea, it is common for the infants to feel listless and inert, and they are often pale. This is a manifestation of dehydration due to insufficient food intake and water loss in respiratory water loss. Physical examination shows the following signs: (1) Flat or reduced affected thoracic site, limited respiratory movement, and suprasternal fossa depression with inspiration. (2) The trachea and apex are displaced to the affected side. (3) Percussion shows slight dullness. (4) Lung auscultation indicates the breath sounds become diminished or disappear. With deep inspiration, coarse crackles can be heard and are important signs of neonatal pulmonary atelectasis. (5) Lung volume diminution can cause diaphragmatic muscle elevation.
2. Lobar atelectasis: Dyspnea may not be obvious, and approximate unilateral atelectasis is a physical sign, albeit to a lesser extent and varies according to the affected lobe. For atelectasis in the upper lobe, the trachea shifts to the affected side, while the heart is not affected; dullness to percussion is limited to the anterior chest area. For atelectasis in the lower lobe, the heart shifts to the affected side, while the tracheal position remains unchanged; dullness to percussion is located at the paravertebral site at the back. For atelectasis in the middle lobe, the physical signs are not obvious and are difficult to investigate.
3. Pulmonary segmental atelectasis: The clinical manifestations are very slight and difficult to identify. They can occur in any pulmonary segment, but they are most rare in the left upper lobe. For congenital heart disease and dilated left pulmonary arteries compressing the left upper lobe of bronchus, left upper lobar atelectasis can be induced.

7.1.3 Disease Course

Obstructive atelectasis can be short or long lasting. For atelectasis induced by a mucus embolism or mucous edema arising from pneumonia, tracheal-bronchiolitis, and meconium aspiration, atelectasis can be resolved with improvement in inflammation. Bilateral or a large area of pulmonary atelectasis can cause death in infants, and it has been reported that the mortality rate from neonatal atelectasis is 11.7%.

7.1.4 Complications [1–5]

The presence of long-term atelectasis can induce secondary infection or worsen the original infection, causing bronchial damage and inflammatory secretion retention, leading to bronchiectasis or emphysema as time passes. It should be noted that atelectasis should be differentiated from lobar pneumonia, pleural effusion, and pulmonary embolism. The diagnosis mainly depends on auxiliary examination.

7.1.5 Auxiliary Examination [1–3]

1. Pulmonary function tests: There are varying degrees of visible reduction in the lung capacity, decreases in the lung compliance, and abnormalities in the ventilation/perfusion ratio, as well as the presence of an arteriovenous shunt and hypoxemia.
2. Chest X-ray examination: The main features are homogeneous dense shadows, which occupy one side, one lobe, or a single pulmonary segment of the lungs. The shadows have no structure, the pulmonary markings disappear, and the lung volume diminishes. In the case of unilateral or a large area of pulmonary atelectasis, intercostal space-narrowing and thoracic cavity diminution are visible. Lower lobar atelectasis forms triangular shadows in the front chest film. These shadows are located between the spine and diaphragmatic muscle. In the lateral chest film, they are located near the lateral chest wall. Upper lobe atelectasis presents as a wedge shape in the anteroposterior and lateral chest film, and the top points to the pulmonary porta. Right middle lobar atelectasis presents as a triangle in the anteroposterior chest film; the bottom is located at the right edge of the heart shadows, and the top points to the lateral side. It presents as a wedge shape in the lateral chest wedge; the bottom is near the anterior chest wall, above the diaphragmatic muscle; and the top points to the posterior upper region.

7.1.6 Treatment [4–7]

For those cases with special causes of atelectasis, the causes should be removed, such as removing the foreign bodies and using antibiotics. The child's position should be changed often; with the child lying in a prone position, atomization is strengthened, and the back is patted so that the secretions are easily eliminated. Tracheal intubation for bronchial lavage and secretion aspiration are effective approaches for neonatal atelectasis treatment, and the treatment can be performed several times a day, as appropriate. However, serious and stubborn bronchial blockage may require bronchoscopic treatment. Bronchoscopic treatment has a good effect on neonatal pulmonary atelectasis, but there are risks, side effects, and complications; units with specific conditions and experienced physicians can implement these treatments.

7.2 Ultrasound Diagnosis of Neonatal Atelectasis

For a long time, the diagnosis of atelectasis has mainly depended on chest X-ray, CT scan, and bronchoscopy. Of these, bronchoscopy is the most reliable method for diagnosing pulmonary atelectasis, but its technical requirements are higher, it is time-consuming, and there is a risk of traumatic occlusion. CT scanning carries a risk of radiation damage, it cannot be performed at the bedside, and it cannot be used in seriously ill infants in the NICU in a timely fashion. Chest X-ray can cause radiation damage, and according to our experience, chest X-ray examination only detects 70% of neonatal pulmonary atelectasis cases. Because of the position of infants for chest X-ray, the lesion site, and transmission direction or the angle influence, it is often difficult to find potential recessive atelectasis. The use of lung ultrasound for diagnosing neonatal lung atelectasis is accurate, it can detect lesions in a timely fashion, it ascertains the lesion severity and range, and it offers an important reference value to guide treatment.

7.2.1 Focal Atelectasis

Atelectasis at the corresponding sites with a relatively large range of lesions in the lung fields found by lung ultrasound examination and verified by transthoracic X-ray. Focal atelectasis has the following characteristics under ultrasound [8, 9]: (1) A large area of consolidation in lesions accompanied by air bronchograms (in severe cases, parallel-arranged linear high echoes are present) or fluid bronchogram (dendrite-shaped distributed linear low echoes are present). (2) The edges of the consolidation areas are regular and clear. (3) The pleural lines are abnormal, and the A-lines disappear. (4) Alveolar-interstitial syndrome is present around the foci. (5) An obvious lung pulse and lung sliding are present under real-time ultrasound. (6) Doppler ultrasound or energy ultrasound indicates pulmonary blood flow in the areas of consolidation.

7.2.2 Occult Lung Atelectasis (OLA)

Refers to potential local atelectasis that is difficult to find by chest X-ray examination and that is common in infants, which makes it difficult to withdraw respirators. The main manifestations under ultrasound are as follows [9]: (1) Local lung consolidation with punctate air bronchograms is present, and the edges of the consolidation areas may be irregular due to the limited range. (2) The pleural line and A-line disappear in the lesion area, while the ultrasound signs in the non-lesion areas remain normal. (3) Under real-time ultrasound, the lung pulse is not obvious, and lung sliding can still occur.

The main ultrasound feature of atelectasis is lung consolidation with bronchograms. Under real-time ultrasound, disappearance of the lung pulse and lung sliding is of some value for further confirmation of the diagnosis of pulmonary atelectasis. When there is a large area of focal atelectasis, lung consolidation becomes significant, the range of consolidation is large, and the air bronchograms are more obvious and may even have a parallel arrangement. For focal atelectasis, the range of consolidation becomes small, and the air bronchogram may not be obvious. Due to the limited lesion range, the lung pulse may be not obvious under real-time ultrasound, and lung sliding may not completely disappear. Because atelectasis is difficult to observe in traditional chest X-ray examination, it is called occult atelectasis. However, lung ultrasound can easily demonstrate these recessive lesions, and this type of atelectasis is common in newborn infants for whom it is difficult to withdraw the ventilator. Possible reasons for the difficulty using traditional X-rays to find this kind of atelectasis are as follows: (1) the influence of the lesion range, the focal range is too small; (2) the influence of the lesion sites and x-line transillumination angles, for lesions at the deep part of the lung field and the posterior back of infants, anteroposterior radiation hides the "occult" lesions; (3) sufficient X-ray transillumination dose; and (4) the influence of patient's spontaneous breathing or assisted ventilation, since newborns cannot cooperate well with technicians to the same degree as infants or adults, imaging may occur during the inspiratory phase.

Disappearance of the pleural line and A-line is a common ultrasound sign, and the scope of disappearance is related to the degree of atelectasis. In the case of a large area of atelectasis, the pleural line and A-line in the entire lung field disappear. In the case of focal atelectasis, the pleural line and A-line only disappear in the lesion sites, and the echoes in the other sites remain normal.

Like atelectasis, the main ultrasound imaging changes of RDS include lung consolidation and air bronchograms. Therefore, it is necessary to correctly differentiate between the two changes. According to our experience, we should learn from the following: (1) The consolidation signs of atelectasis are seen in the recovery period of primary lung diseases, and the above signs are common in the acute stage of RDS. (2) In the case of atelectasis, air bronchograms often present in a linear parallel arrangement, while RDS often has a punctiform arrangement without regularities, which is associated with the degree and scope of consolidation. (3) For RDS, pleural effusion and "white lung" changes can be seen, and such signs can be observed with atelectasis.

The main ultrasound manifestation of neonate infectious pneumonia is a large area of lung consolidation with air bronchograms. However, for pneumonia, the borders of the consolidation areas are irregular, the consolidation areas with varying sizes and ranges are present in different lung fields of the same liver, and the air bronchogram is dynamic (Figs. 7.1–7.19).

We stated that all the pictures or ultrasound images included in the chapter were taken from the Army General Hospital of the Chinese PLA and Beijing Chaoyang District Maternal and Child Health Care Hospital; the related studies were approved by both the committee of the Army General Hospital and Chaoyang District Maternal and Child Healthcare Hospital.

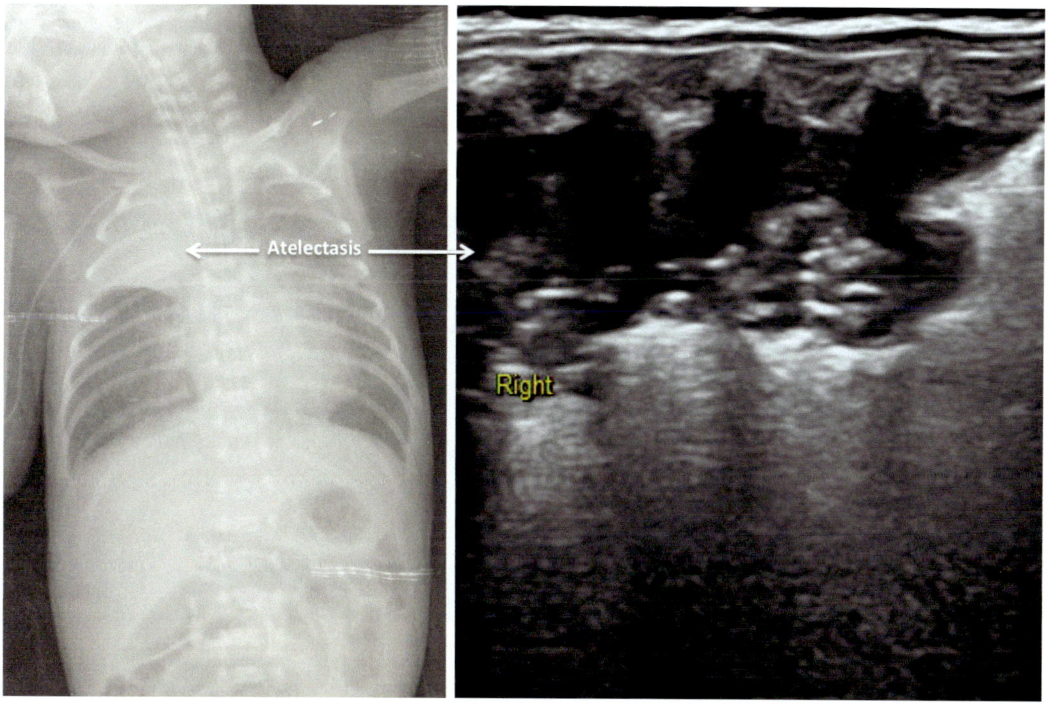

Fig. 7.1 Ultrasound signs of atelectasis. Infant with a gestational age of 29 weeks and a birth weight of 890 g who was diagnosed with respiratory distress syndrome on admission. Lung ultrasound showed a large area of consolidation, with clearly demarcated borders and air bronchograms (hyperechogenic lines in the area of consolidation) and fluid bronchograms (hypoechogenic lines in the area of consolidation) in the upper right lung. Chest radiograph (CXR) findings confirmed atelectasis in the area of consolidation

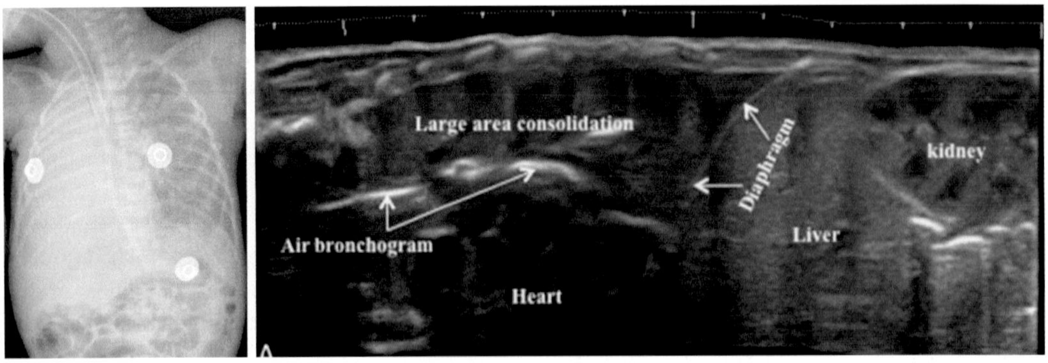

Fig. 7.2 Ultrasound signs of atelectasis. Infant with a gestational age of 30^{+4} weeks and a birth weight of 1480 g who was delivered by cesarean section. The infant had been treated with mechanical ventilation for 14 days because of respiratory distress syndrome and ventilator-associated pneumonia and then had a relapse of respiratory distress soon after weaning from ventilation. A bedside lung ultrasound showed a large area of consolidation in the right lung with obvious air and fluid bronchograms. The echogenicity of the consolidated lung tissue was similar to that of the adjacent liver tissue, which confirmed complete right lung atelectasis that was observed by chest X-ray

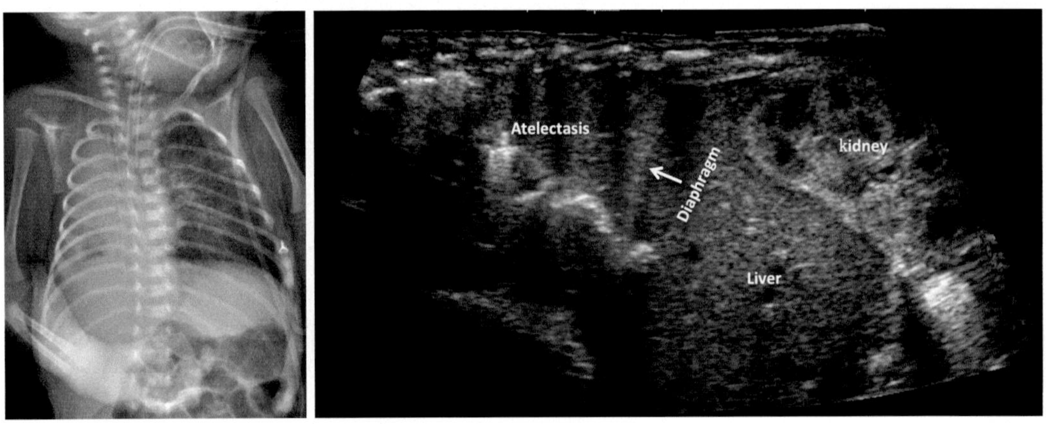

Fig. 7.3 Ultrasound signs of atelectasis. Infant with a gestational age of 29^{+1} weeks and a birth weight of 890 g who was diagnosed with pneumonia on admission. Lung ultrasound showed a large area of consolidation with clearly demarcated borders and air bronchograms in the upper right lung. CXR confirmed atelectasis in the area of consolidation

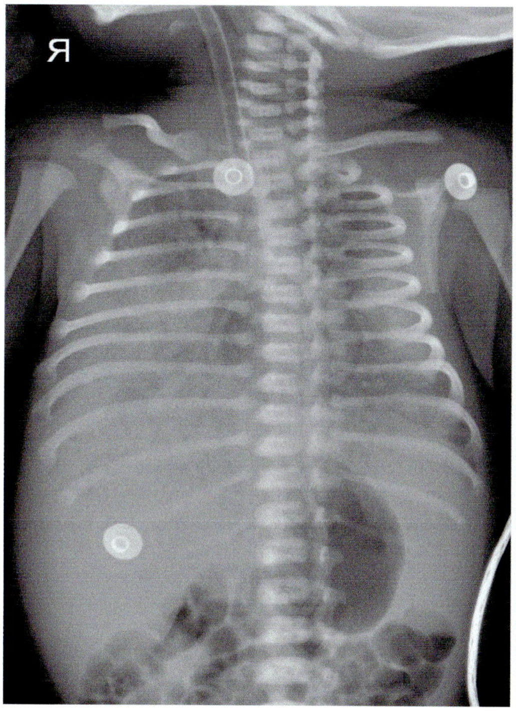

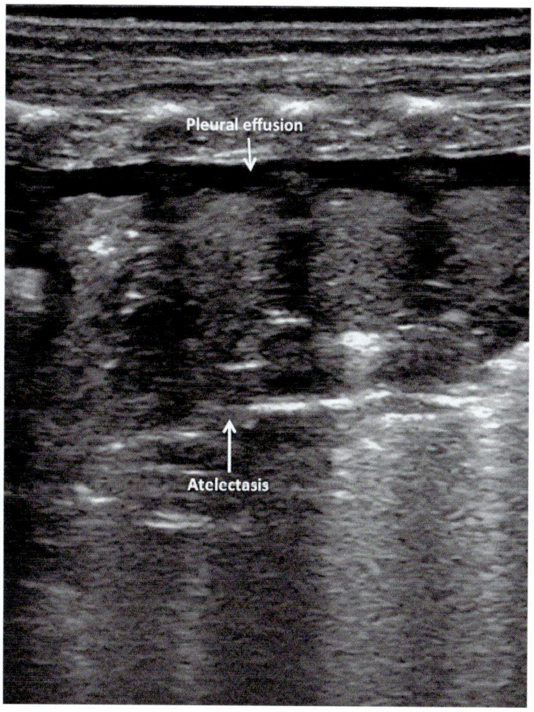

Fig. 7.4 Ultrasound signs of atelectasis. Infant with a gestational age of 38^{+1} weeks and a birth weight of 3020 g who was born via vaginal delivery. The patient was admitted to the hospital due to intrauterine infectious pneumonia. Multiple sputum cultures indicated *Klebsiella pneumoniae*, and the patient was given mechanical ventilation for treatment of dyspnea. Two months after birth, the patient continued to rely on the respirator, which could not be withdrawn. Lung ultrasound reveals a large area of consolidation in the right upper lung field accompanied by air bronchograms; real-time ultrasound shows the disappearance of lung sliding as well as the A-line and consolidation pleural line, and chest X-ray examination confirms the diagnosis of atelectasis. A small amount of pleural effusion can be seen in this patient

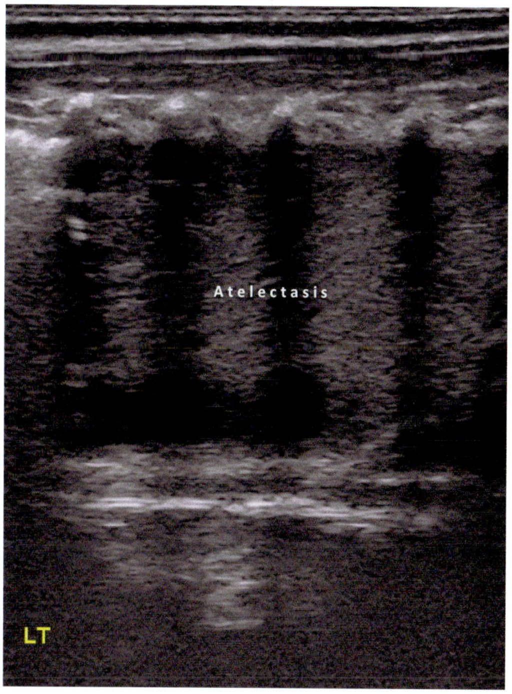

Fig. 7.5 Ultrasound signs of atelectasis. Infant with a gestational age of 28^{+6} weeks and a birth weight of 1450 g. The patient was admitted due to RDS, and the machine was withdrawn after 18 days of respirator treatment. However, after the machine was withdrawn, dyspnea remained obvious. A back longitudinal scan shows a large area of consolidation in the right lower lung, which is very close to the echoes of the adjacent liver tissues accompanied by bronchograms; disappearance of A-lines and pleural lines and an obvious lung pulse with disappearance of lung sliding are seen under real-time ultrasound

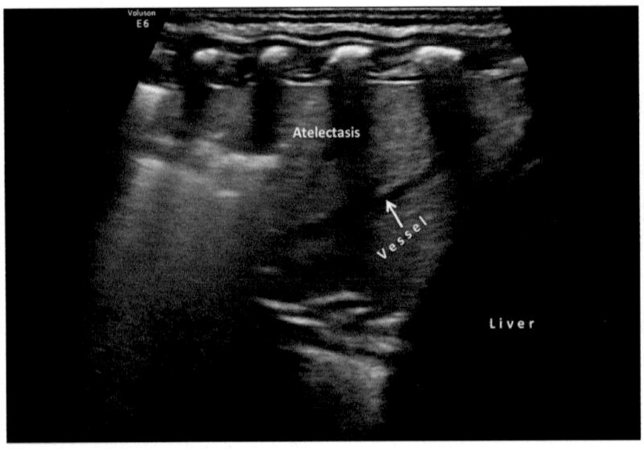

Fig. 7.6 Right lower pulmonary atelectasis. Infant with a gestational age of 37^{+5} weeks and a birth weight of 3245 g who was born by cesarean section without asphyxia; the infant had dyspnea after birth, and dense moist rales were heard in both lungs. Arterial blood gas analysis was as follows: pH 7.26, $PaCO_2$ 48 mmHg, PaO_2 67 mmHg, and BE-5 mmol/L. Routine blood test indicated the following: WBC 50 × 10^9/L, proportion of stab nuclei of 3%, N% 76%, PLT 22 × 10^9/L, and CRP 76 mg/L. Chest X-ray confirmed there were changes consistent with pneumonia. At 12 days after birth, lung ultrasound showed consolidation in the right lung field and disappearance of the pleural line, suggesting the presence of atelectasis. The arrow in the figure indicates that the linear low echoes are the pulmonary vessels and the difference with the fluid bronchogram should be noted

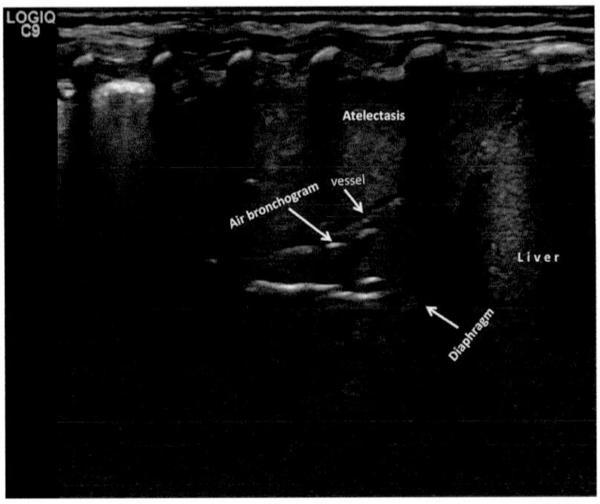

Fig. 7.7 Atelectasis. Infant with a gestational age of 37^{+3} weeks and a birth weight of 3500 g who was born by cesarean section. The patient was admitted due to intrauterine infectious pneumonia and was treated with mechanical ventilation. However, the recovery was not smooth. At 9 days after birth, lung ultrasound showed lung consolidation over three intercostals in the right lung accompanied by air bronchograms, while the pleural line was blurred and the lung pulse was visible under the real-time ultrasound, suggesting a large area of atelectasis

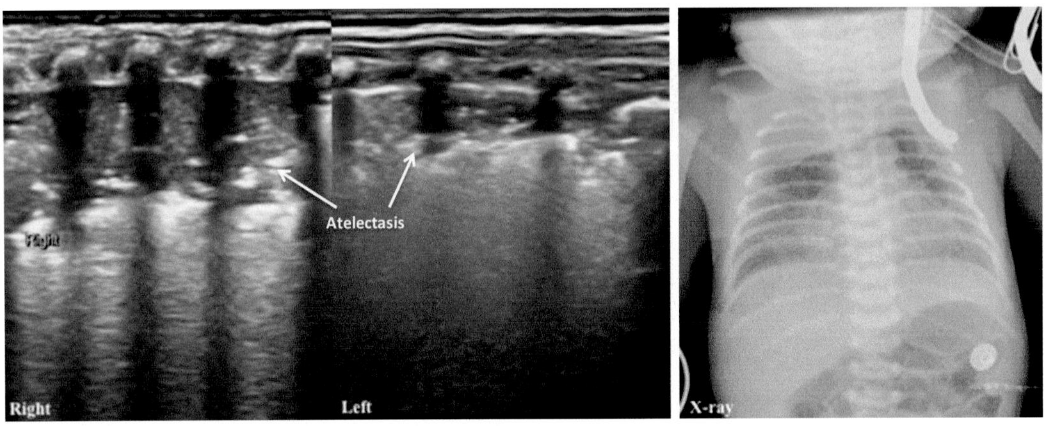

Fig. 7.8 Atelectasis of both lungs. Infant with a gestational age of 36^{+6} weeks and a birth weight of 2850 g who was born via vaginal delivery without asphyxia at birth after the occurrence of PROM 41 h prior. Dyspnea occurred shortly after birth. At admission, there were dense and moist rales in both lungs, a fever gradually occurred, and a diagnosis of pneumonia was made. After treatment, the body temperature gradually dropped, but dyspnea remained obvious. At 12 days after birth, lung ultrasound showed a large area of lung consolidation with air bronchograms (*arrow*); the right manifestation was particularly serious, the pleural line was blurred or disappeared, the A-line disappeared, and the transthoracic X-ray examination confirmed the diagnosis of atelectasis of both lungs

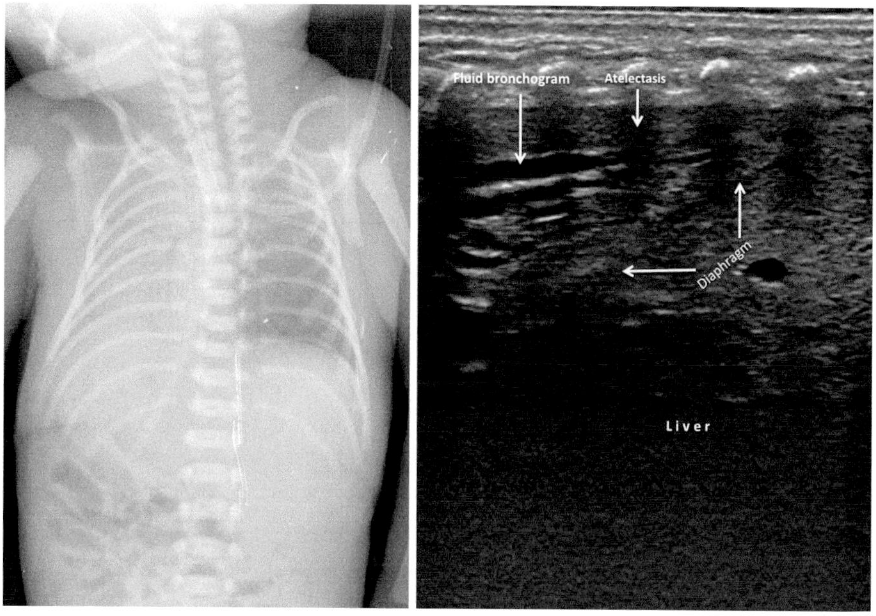

Fig. 7.9 Complete right lung atelectasis. Chest X-ray showed complete right lung atelectasis. Lung ultrasound showed a large area of consolidation with regular margins (atelectasis) in the right lung field. Under real-time ultrasound, consolidated lung movement could be seen with his respiratory movement (Video 7.1)

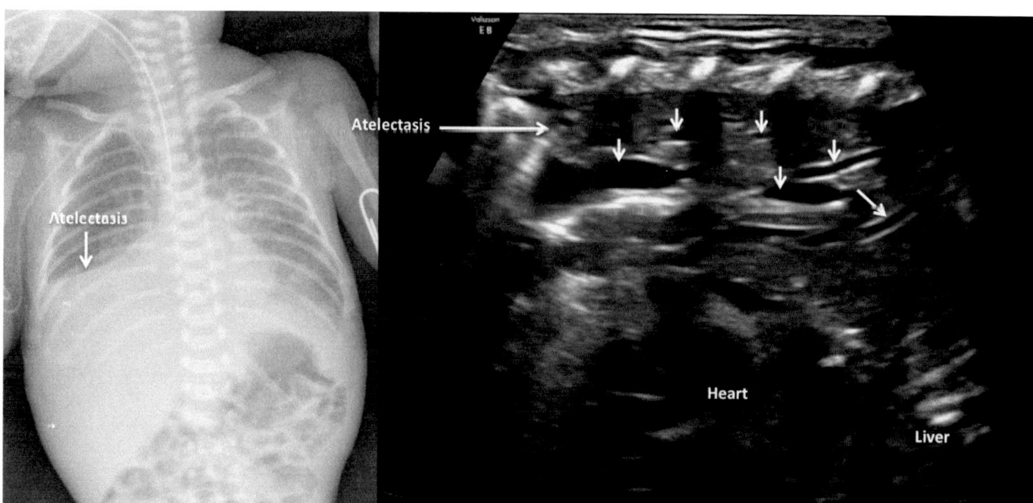

Fig. 7.10 Right lower lung atelectasis with fluid bronchograms. Chest X-ray and ultrasound showing a large area of atelectasis in the right lower lung field. Tubular anechoic areas in the consolidation region suggest that the bronchi are filled with liquid (*arrow*), and the bronchial wall is hyperechoic, which is called a fluid bronchogram. Lung consolidation with a fluid bronchogram is relatively rare, but it is one of the characteristic changes in serious lung consolidation

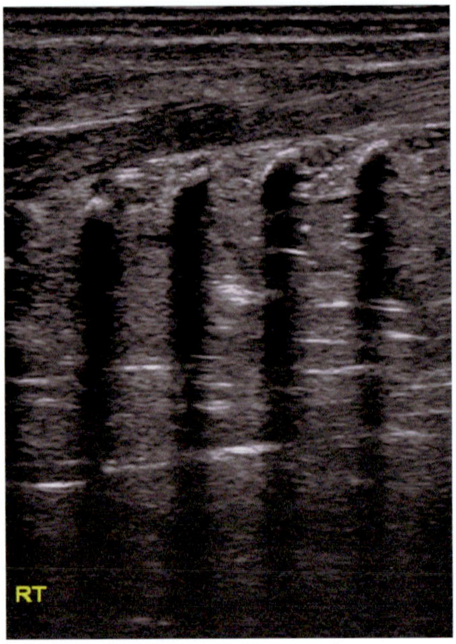

Fig. 7.11 Parallel air bronchograms in severe atelectasis. Parallel air bronchograms were often seen in patients with severe atelectasis, as in this patient who had consolidation of the whole right lung

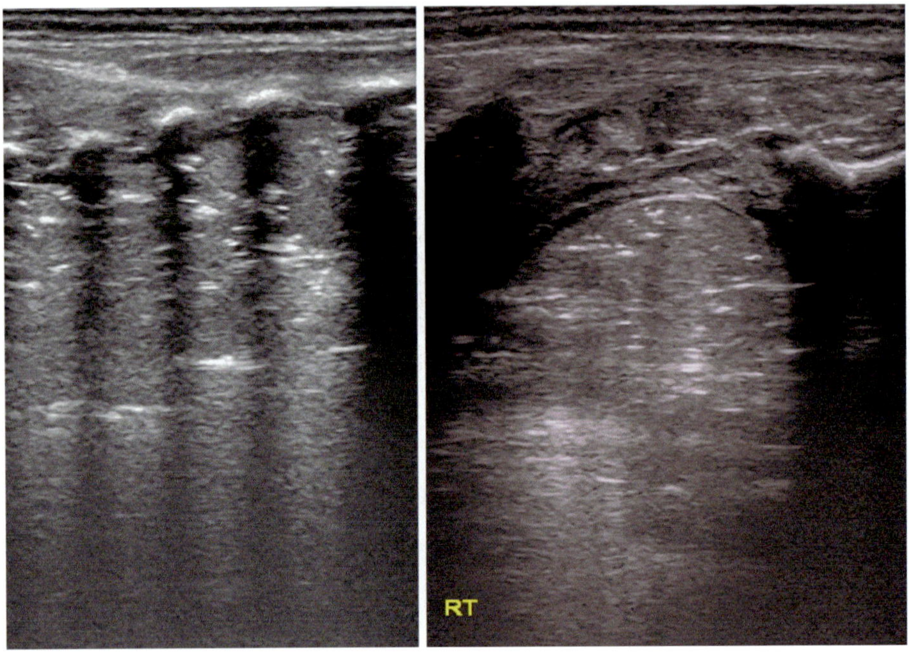

Fig. 7.12 Dynamic air bronchograms in severe atelectasis. Significant air bronchograms can be seen in this atelectasis patient (left, the probe is perpendicular to the ribs, and right, the probe is parallel to the ribs). Under real-time ultrasound, the air bronchograms can be found moving with respiration, and this movement is known as dynamic air bronchograms (Videos 7.2 and 7.3)

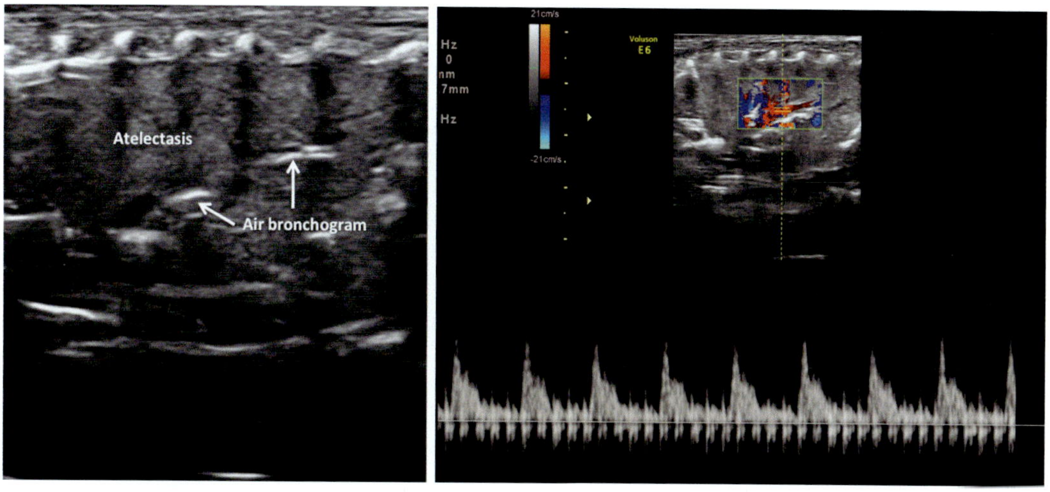

Fig. 7.13 Blood flow within areas of atelectasis. Infant with a gestational age of 25^{+3} weeks and a birth weight of 730 g who was born vaginally via induced premature labor after PROM for 11 days. Test tube baby Apgar scores were 7–7–7 points at 1–5–10 min. The patient was admitted due to premature labor and dyspnea. Routine blood test results were as follows: WBC 55 × 10^9/L, proportion of myelocytes of 4%, proportion of metagranulocytes of 8%, proportion of stab cells of 9%, proportion of neutrophils of 59%, PLT 146 × 10^9/L, and CRP 90.0 mg/L. The diagnosis was intrauterine infectious pneumonia of the newborn. At 4 days after birth, lung ultrasound shows right lower pulmonary lobar consolidation with slight air bronchograms. The lung parenchymal echo was adjacent to the liver echo, and the color Doppler ultrasound shows a lung arterial blood supply and blood flow frequency spectrum within the pulmonary tissues of consolidation areas. Real-time ultrasound shows that consolidation tissues move with heart pulsation, namely, the lung pulse

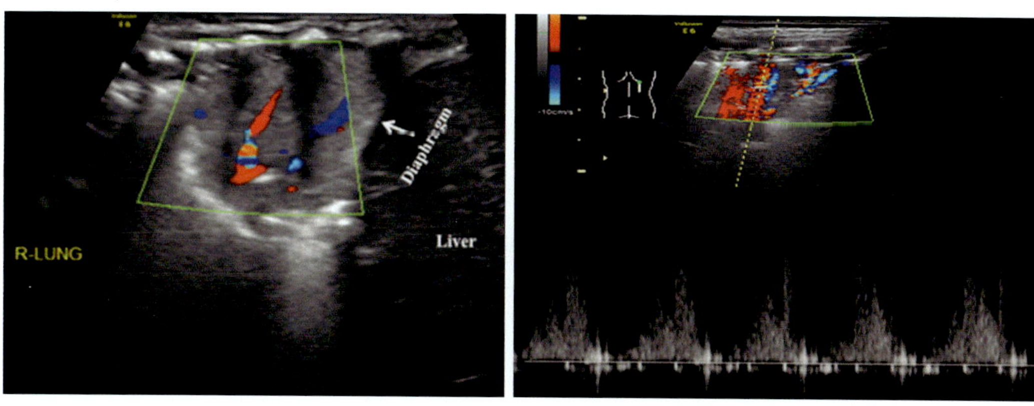

Fig. 7.14 Atelectasis and blood supply. Infant with a gestational age of 32 weeks and a birth weight of 2050 g who was born by cesarean section. The patient was admitted due to pneumonia. At 1 week after birth, lung ultrasound showed a relatively large range of consolidation areas in the right lower lung, a visible air bronchogram and disappearance of pleural and A-lines, indicating the presence of atelectasis. Color Doppler ultrasound shows a rich blood supply within the consolidation areas. The right figure shows the blood supply status within consolidation areas under real-time Doppler monitoring

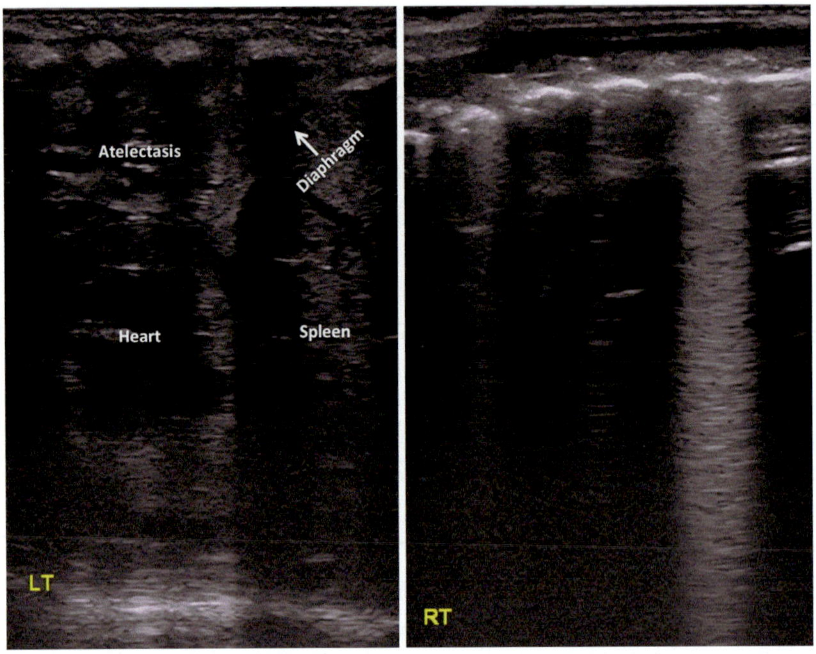

Fig. 7.15 Lung pulse in atelectasis patients. Severe atelectasis in the left lung. Under real-time ultrasound, we can see the movement of a lung with atelectasis with the heart pulse; this movement is called the lung pulse (Video 7.4)

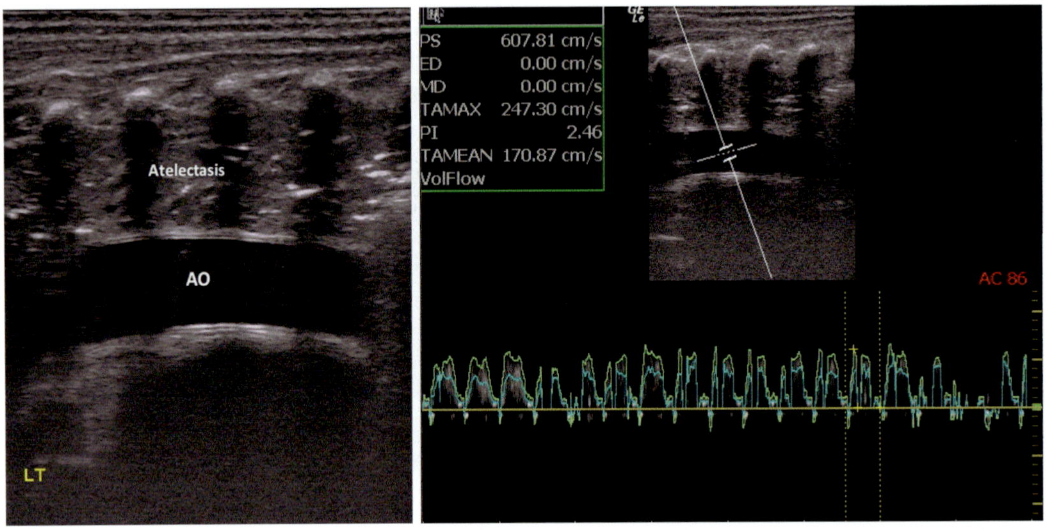

Fig. 7.16 Lung pulse in atelectasis patients. Lung ultrasound showing a large area atelectasis with air and fluid bronchograms in the left lung. One blood vessel could be seen clearly under ultrasound, which was confirmed by Doppler ultrasonography. Under real-time ultrasound, a significant lung pulse can be seen (Video 7.5)

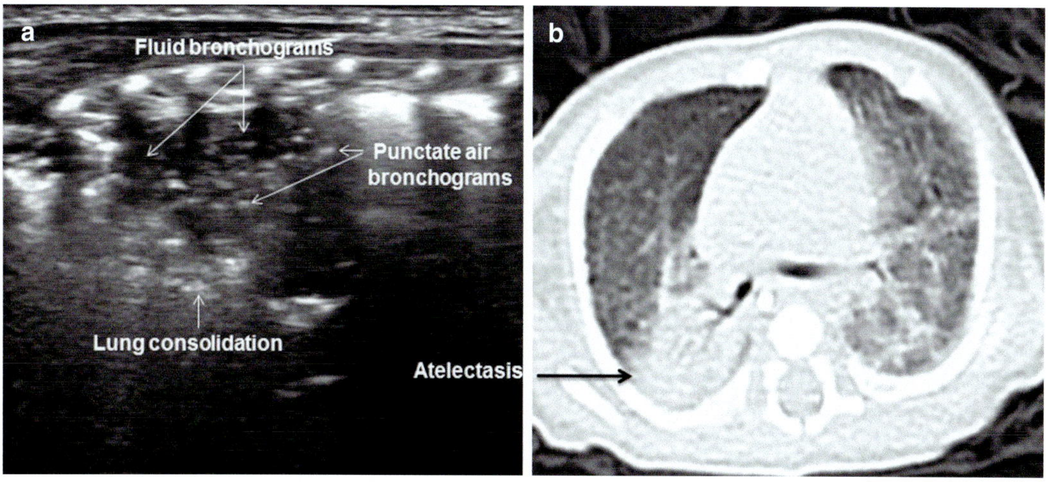

Fig. 7.17 The ultrasound appearance of occult lung atelectasis (OLA). Infant with a gestational age of 29^{+1} weeks and a birth weight of 890 g who was born via vaginal delivery. Diagnosed as RDS on admission and still dependent on oxygen at 5 months after birth. Lung ultrasound showed upper right lung consolidation with punctate air bronchograms and fluid bronchograms. The lower right lung field demonstrates interstitial syndrome (**a**). While the chest X-ray has no abnormal findings, the chest CT scan confirms the presence of upper right lung atelectasis (**b**)

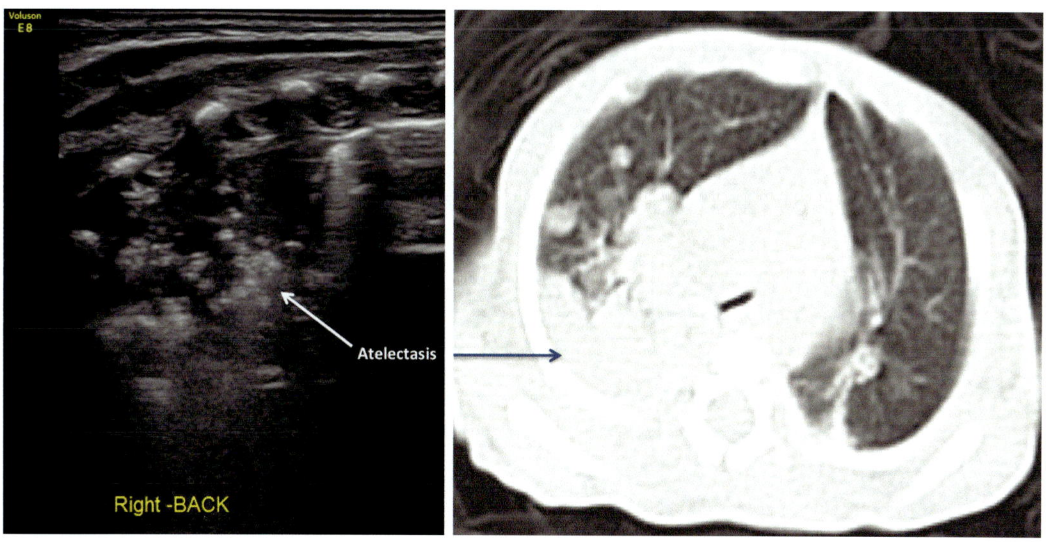

Fig. 7.18 The ultrasound appearance of OLA. Infant at a gestational age of 37^{+6} weeks and a birth weight of 3880 g who was born via cesarean delivery. Diagnosed as MAS on admission and treated with mechanical ventilation for 7 days. The baby was re-ventilated because of ongoing breathing difficulty after withdrawing ventilator support for 4 days. The baby required mechanical ventilation for another 3 days. The baby again experienced distress when the ventilator was withdrawn. Bedside lung ultrasound showed focal upper right lung field lung consolidation with air bronchograms as well as disappearance of pleural and A-lines. The lower right lung field has a normal appearance ("black" lung field; pleural and A-lines are clearly present). At the same time, the chest X-ray has no abnormal findings, while the chest CT scan confirms the presence of upper right lung atelectasis

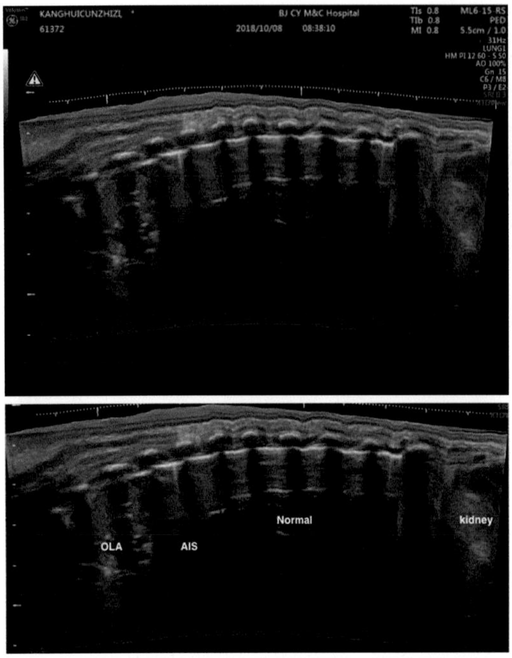

Fig. 7.19 OLA (volume panorama mode). A OLA patient. Ultrasound (volume panorama) showed OLA, AIS and normal lung area in sequence

References

1. Peroni DG, Boner AL. Atelectasis: mechanisms, diagnosis and management. Paediatr Respir Rev. 2000;1(3):274–8.
2. Johnston C, Carvalho WB. Atelectasis: mechanisms, diagnosis and treatment in the pediatric patient. Rev Assoc Med Bras. 2008;54(5):455–60.
3. Nakos G, Tsangaris H, Liokatis S, et al. Ventilator-associated pneumonia and atelectasis: evaluation through bronchoalveolar lavage fluid analysis. Intensive Care Med. 2003;29:555–63.
4. Westhoff M, Freitag L. Surfactant treatment of complete lobar atelectasis after exacerbation of bronchial asthma by infection. Pneumologie. 2001;55:130–4.
5. Schindler MB. Treatment of atelectasis: where is the evidence? Crit Care. 2005;9(4):341–2.
6. Bar-Zohar D, Sivan Y. The yield of flexible fiberoptic bronchoscopy in pediatric intensive care patients. Chest. 2004;126:1353–9.
7. Zhang DJ, Zhao DY, Liang H, et al. Application of flexible bronchoscopy in diagnosis and treatment of 104 children with pulmonary atelectasis. Zhonghua Er Ke Za Zhi. 2010;48(10):767–70.
8. Lichtenstein DA, Lascols N, Prin S, et al. The "lung pulse": an early ultrasound sign of complete atelectasis. Intensive Care Med. 2003;29:2187–92.
9. Liu J, Chen SW, Liu F, et al. The diagnosis of neonatal pulmonary atelectasis using lung ultrasonography. Chest. 2015;147(4):1013–9.

Pulmonary Hemorrhage of the Newborn

8

Jing Liu and Erich Sorantin

8.1 Pulmonary Hemorrhage

Pulmonary hemorrhage of the newborn (PHN) is a common severe and critical disease in newborn infants, exhibiting complicated etiologies, rapid progression, and a high mortality rate [1, 2]. It was reported that the incidence rate of PHN was 1–12‰ of live births, increasing to 50‰ in infants with high-risk factors [3]. The common risk factors included premature birth, intrauterine growth restriction (IUGR), patent ductus arteriosus (PDA), severe birth asphyxia, hypoxia, oxygen toxicity, disseminated intravascular coagulation (DIC), RDS, MAS, hypotension, severe infection or sepsis, polycythemia, mechanical ventilation, multiple births, male gender, and surfactant therapy [1]. We observed that the primary causes of PHN were severe intrauterine infection (33.3%), severe birth asphyxia (21.1%), and RDS (21.1%), accounting for more than 75% of the patients. MAS and severe postnatal infection accounted for 25% of these patients. PHN often occurred within the first several days after birth. In this study, 71.4% of the cases developed PHN within several hours to 24 h after birth, 80.4% developed PHN within 3 days of life, 89.5% developed PHN within 7 days of life, and only 10.5% developed PHN between 1 and 2 weeks after birth, meaning that nearly 90% of the NPH cases occurred within the first week of life.

Until recent years, the mortality of NPH was as high as 50%. The survival of infants was affected by several factors contributing to a long-term poor prognosis. For example, the incidence of nerve sensory disturbance doubled in severe NPH patients; the incidence of bronchopulmonary dysplasia, cerebral palsy, and cognitive delay increased 2.5 times in premature infants with NPH; and the incidence of seizure associated with periventricular leukomalacia also increased significantly [1]. Recently, mortality decreased significantly with the development of new treatment methods [4–6].

The key protocol for decreasing NPH mortality is based on early, quick, and accurate diagnosis. For a long time, the diagnosis of PHN was based on medical history, typical clinical presentation, and chest X-ray examination. Although chest X-ray is non-specific, it is usually necessary for the diagnosis of PHN often manifesting as fluffy opacities, focal ground-glass opacities, or even "white-out" in severe patients. Lung ultrasound is not usually performed in cases of suspected

Electronic Supplementary Material The online version of this chapter (https://doi.org/10.1007/978-94-024-1549-0_8) contains supplementary material, which is available to authorized users.

J. Liu (✉)
Department of Neonatology and NICU, Beijing Chaoyang District Maternal and Child Health Care Hospital, Beijing, China

E. Sorantin
Division of Pediatric Radiology, Department of Radiology, Medical University Graz, Graz, Austria

J. Liu et al. (eds.), *Neonatal Lung Ultrasonography*, https://doi.org/10.1007/978-94-024-1549-0_8

PHN. Therefore, we investigated the diagnostic value of lung ultrasound for PHN. Through the systemic observation of lung ultrasonic characteristics of PHN patients, we observed that lung ultrasound can accurately diagnose NPH. This method was also useful for dynamic observation and timely understanding of the changes of pulmonary lesions and thus was helpful in guiding treatment and improving prognosis.

8.2 Ultrasound Diagnosis of Pulmonary Hemorrhage

According to the results of this study, we found that the major ultrasonic characteristics of PHN were the following [7]:

1. Shred sign: It is characterized as the border between the aerated lung and consolidated lung not being sharp [8]. The shred sign is the most common ultrasonic sign of PHN, occurring in more than 90% of the patients. The shred sign was the main ultrasonic finding in mild PHN patients or within the lung on the side with mild bleeding. In addition, the shred sign was often found at the edge of large areas of consolidation.
2. Lung consolidation with an air bronchogram: This was one of the most common ultrasonic signs of PHN, seen in more than 80% of the patients. We think that the reasons for consolidation were mainly related to the original lung disease, the lung bleeding itself, or the secretions blocking the trachea and bronchus.
3. Pleural effusion: This is another common sign of PHN, occurring in more than 85% of the PHN cases. Pleural effusion can be observed in one or both sides of the thorax but is often seen on the side with more severe bleeding in the lung. The fluid amount was associated with the original disease and/or the degree of bleeding. The fluid was confirmed as bleeding by thoracocentesis. Severe cases were due to the destruction of red blood cells, and fibrous protein depositions resulted in the formation of fibrous cord-like floating objects. These floating objects could be observed with fluid movement under real-time ultrasound (avi-1).
4. Pulmonary atelectasis: This was seen in one third of the patients. In addition to lung consolidation, atelectasis was mainly related to the original lung disease, such as pneumonia, RDS, or MAS, while lung bleeding itself or the secretions blocking the trachea and bronchus were also associated with these pathogenic findings.
5. Abnormal pleural lines and A-line disappearance: Both of these signs were the most common and non-specific ultrasonic findings of PHN.
6. AIS: In some cases with mild bleeding, or in the acute stages of some cases with severe bleeding, AIS was the main manifestation.

Lung ultrasound for the diagnosis of PHN had high sensitivity and specificity. According to the results of our study, the shred sign, which had a sensitivity of 91.2% and a specificity of 100%, was especially helpful for diagnosing PHN [7] (Figs. 8.1, 8.2, 8.3, 8.4, 8.5, 8.6, 8.7, and 8.8).

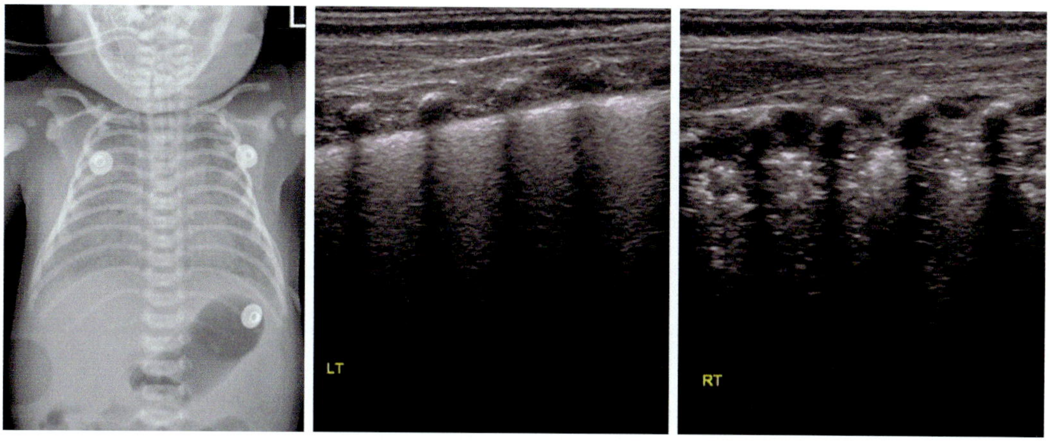

Fig. 8.1 Shred sign was the most common ultrasonic sign of NPH. The baby was the product of a G_1P_1 mother, gestational age 41 weeks, admitted to the NICU because of lung bleeding. The chest X-ray had high density cloudy shadows in the right lung field. The lung ultrasound manifested with AIS and a thickened and fuzzy pleura in the left lung, while the right lung showed consolidation with an air bronchogram and shred sign

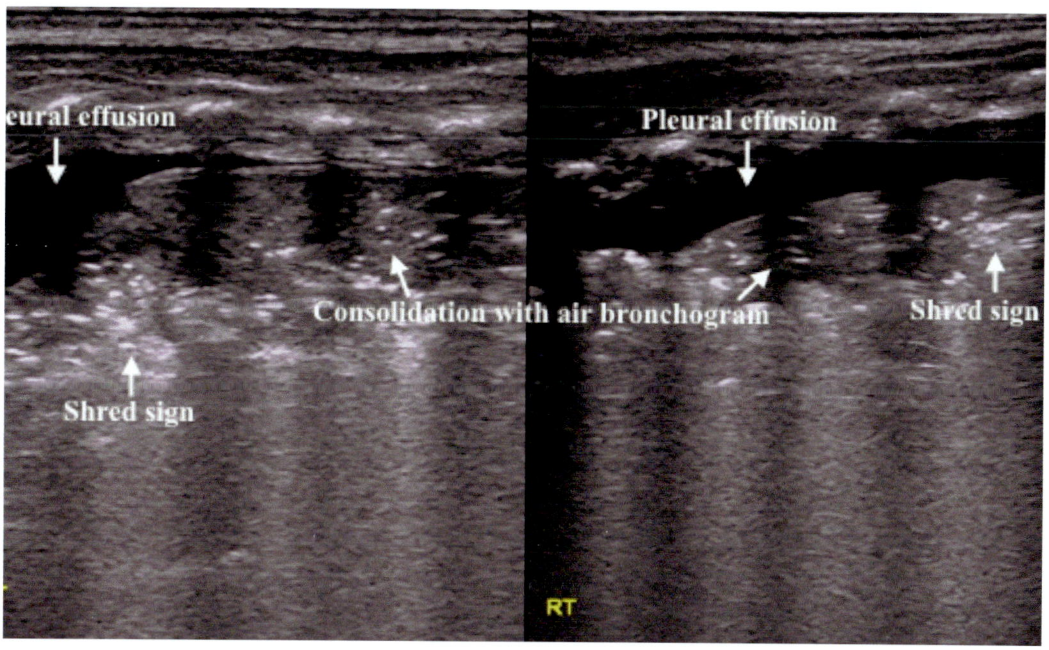

Fig. 8.2 Ultrasonic findings in a severe NPH case. The baby was the product of a G_3P_1 mother with a gestational age of 37^{+1} weeks, delivered via cesarean section with a birth weight of 4600 g. The baby was admitted to the NICU because of NPH caused by MAS. The lung ultrasound showed a large area of lung consolidation with an air bronchogram, a shred sign, an absent pleural line, and A-lines on both sides of the lungs, as well as pleural effusion in the right lung

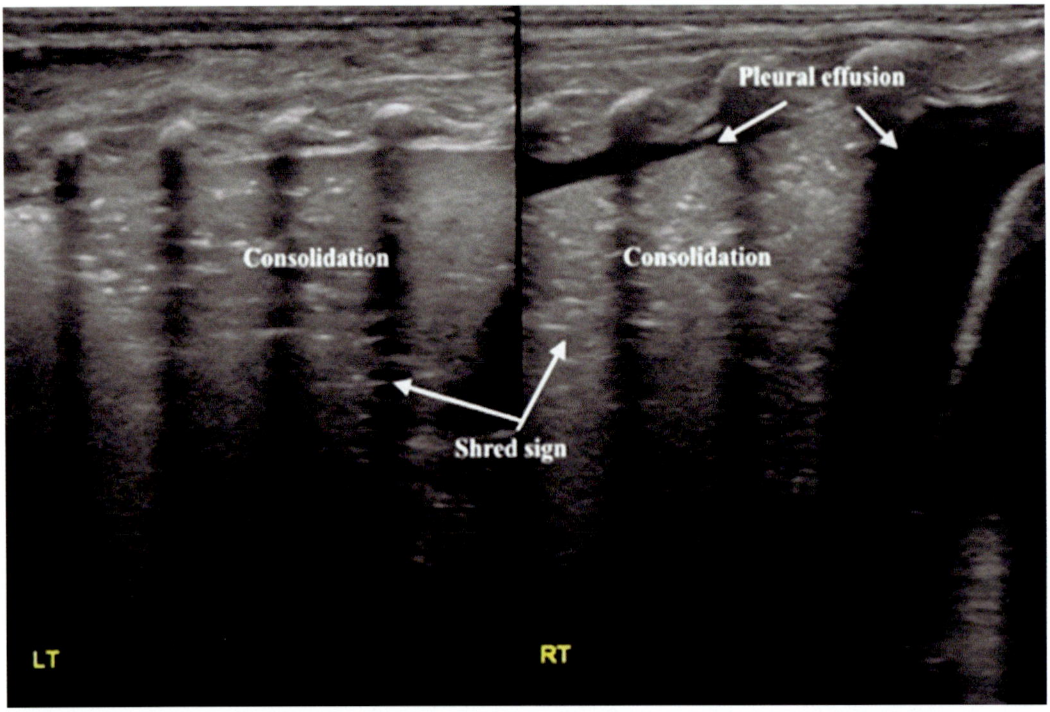

Fig. 8.3 Ultrasonic findings in a severe NPH case. The baby was G_1P_1 with a gestational age of 38^{+6} weeks, delivered by cesarean section with a birth weight of 3345 g. The baby was admitted to the NICU because of NPH caused by severe birth asphyxia. The lung ultrasound showed a large area of lung consolidation with an air bronchogram, a shred sign at the edge of consolidation, a disappeared pleural line, A-lines in both sides of the lungs, and pleural effusion in the right lung (confirmed as bleeding by thoracocentesis)

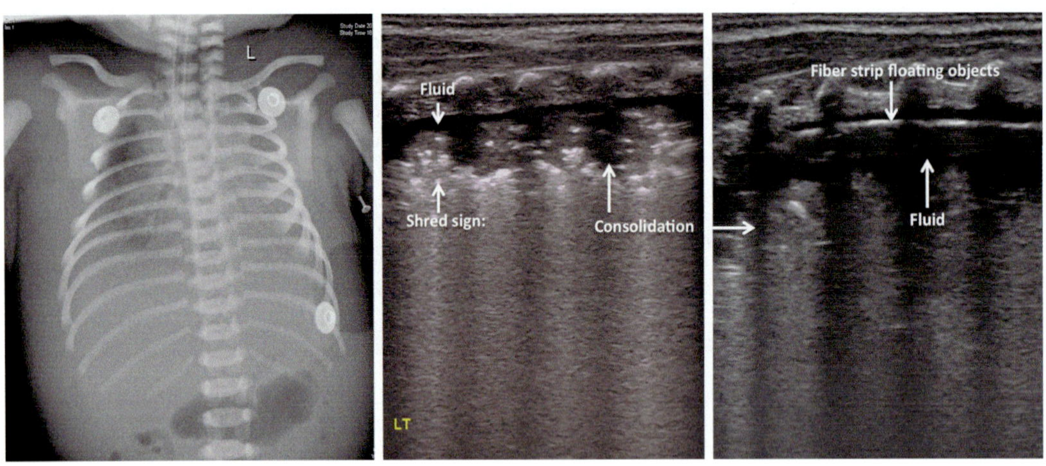

Fig. 8.4 Ultrasonic findings in a severe NPH case. The baby was G_1P_1 with gestational age of 39^{+6} weeks delivered vaginally with a birth weight of 3180 g. The baby was admitted to the NICU because of NPH caused by severe intrauterine infection. The lung ultrasound showed a large area of lung consolidation with an air bronchogram, a shred sign at the edge of consolidation, pleural effusion in both sides of the lungs (confirmed as bleeding by thoracocentesis), and a disappeared pleural line and A-lines. It was observed that there was fibrous protein deposition in the formation of fibrous cord-like floating objects with fluid movement under real-time ultrasound (Video 8.1)

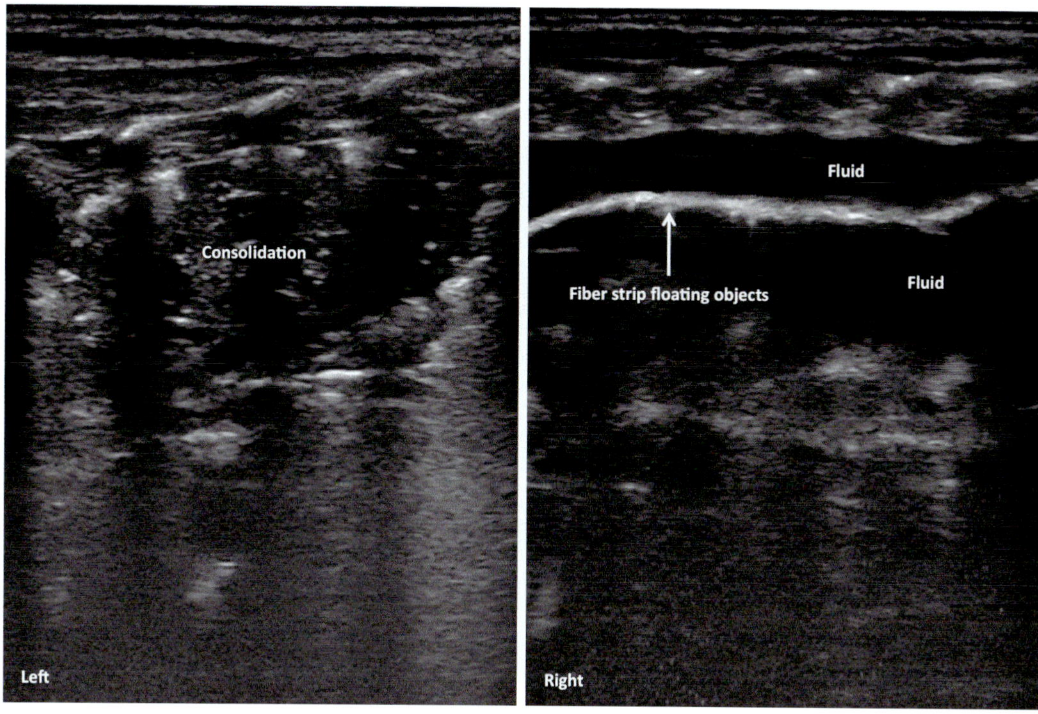

Fig. 8.5 Ultrasonic findings in a severe NPH case. The baby was G_2P_1 with gestational age 33^{+3} weeks, delivered vaginally with a birth weight of 2160 g. The baby was admitted to the NICU because of NPH. The lung ultrasound showed a large area of consolidation in the left lung and large amount of pleural effusion in the right chest (confirmed as bleeding by thoracocentesis). It was observed that there was fibrous protein deposition in the formation of fibrous cord-like floating objects

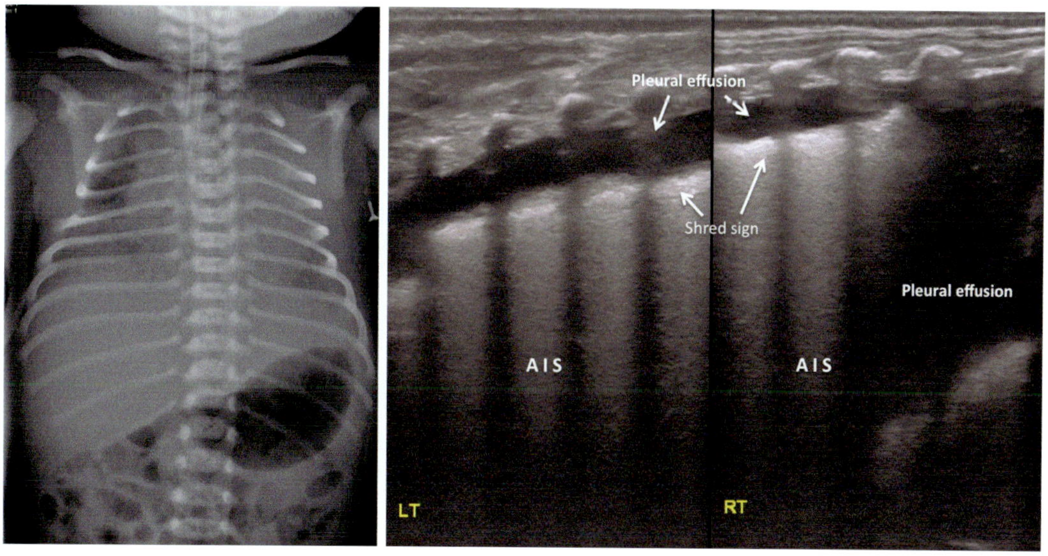

Fig. 8.6 Pleural effusion can be the main ultrasonic findings of NPH patients. The baby was G_3P_1 with gestational age of 39 weeks, delivery by cesarean section with a birth weight of 3200 g. The baby was admitted to the NICU because of NPH. The chest X-ray showed nearly "white lung" with pleural effusion in bilateral chest (more significantly on the right). The lung ultrasound showed significant pleural effusion on both sides of the chest (more severe in the right chest). The fluid was confirmed as bleeding by thoracocentesis. The other findings were AIS and mild shred signs

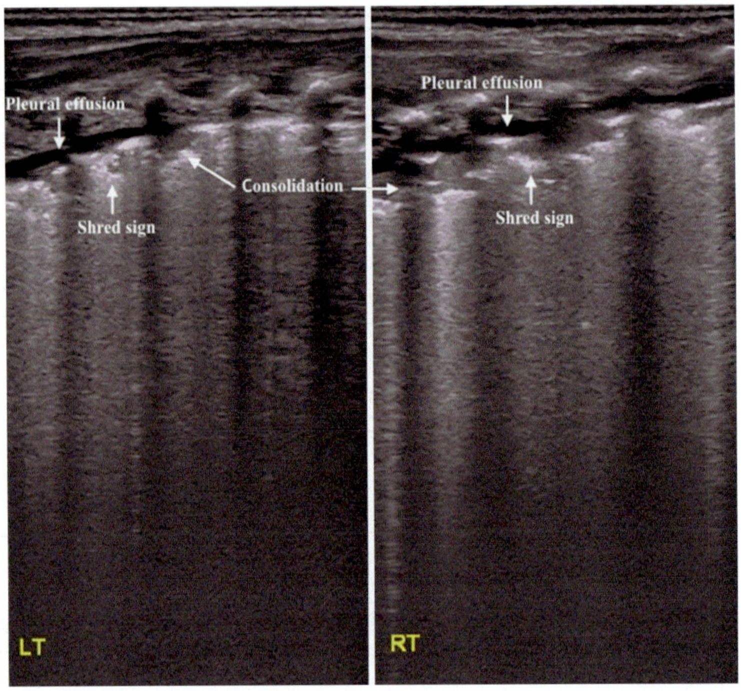

Fig. 8.7 Ultrasonic findings in a mild NPH case. The baby was G_2P_1 with gestational age of 38^+ weeks, delivered vaginally with a birth weight of 3070 g. The baby was admitted to the NICU because of **NPH** caused by severe asphyxia. The ultrasound showed small consolidation with an air bronchogram under the pleural line and a shred sign at the edge of consolidation, as well as an abnormality of the pleural line, an absent A-line, and a small amount of pleural effusion

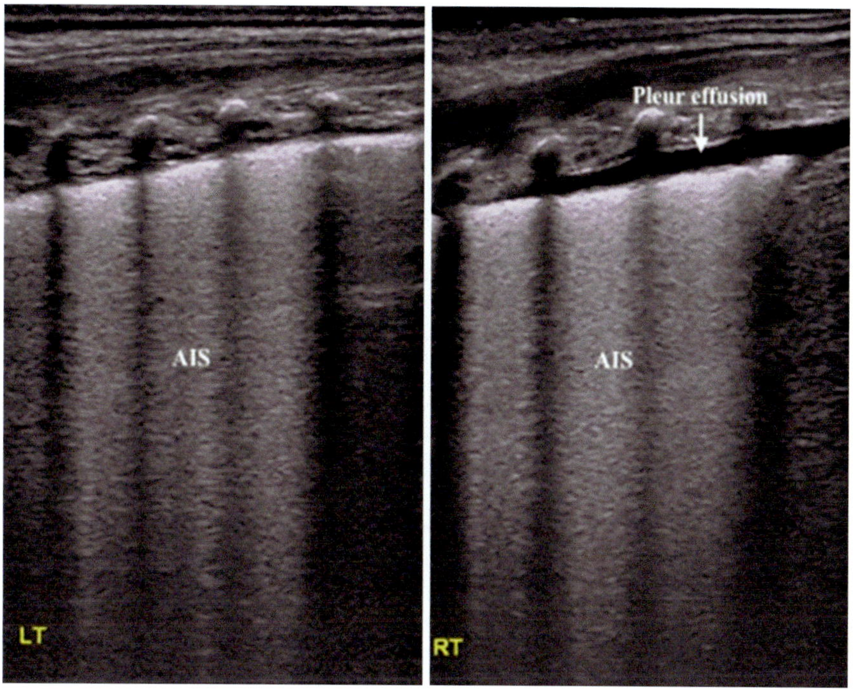

Fig. 8.8 Ultrasonic findings in the acute stages of NPH. The baby was G_1P_1 with gestational age of 39^{+5} weeks, delivered vaginally with a birth weight of 3370 g. The baby was admitted to the NICU with a diagnosis of RDS. NPH was diagnosed 10 h after admission to the hospital when the lung ultrasound showed AIS, a fuzzy pleural line, and disappeared A-lines, as well as a small pleural effusion in the right side of the thorax

References

1. Zahr RA, Ashfaq A, Marron-Corwin M. Neonatal pulmonary hemorrhage. NeoReviews. 2012;13(5):e302.
2. Shi Y, Zhao J, Tang S, Pan F, Liu L, et al. Effect of hemocoagulase for prevention of pulmonary hemorrhage in critical newborns on mechanical ventilation: a randomized controlled trial. Indian Pediatr. 2008;45(3):199–202.
3. Berger TM, Allred EN, Van Marter LJ. Antecedents of clinically significant pulmonary hemorrhage among newborn infants. J Perinatol. 2000;20(5):295–300.
4. AlKharfy TM. High-frequency ventilation in the management of very-low-birth-weight infants with pulmonary hemorrhage. Am J Perinatol. 2004;21(1):19–26.
5. Lodha A, Kamaluddeen M, Akierman A, Amin H. Role of hemocoagulase in pulmonary hemorrhage in preterm infants: a systematic review. Indian J Pediatr. 2011;78(7):838–44.
6. Shi Y, Tang S, Li H, Zhao J, Pan F. New treatment of neonatal pulmonary hemorrhage with hemocoagulase in addition to mechanical ventilation. Biol Neonate. 2005;88(2):118–21.
7. Ren XL, Fu W, Liu J, et al. Lung ultrasonography to diagnose pulmonary hemorrhage of the newborn. J Matern Fetal Neonatal Med. 2017;30(21):2601–6.
8. Touw HRW, Tuinman PR, Gelissen HPMM, et al. Lung ultrasound: routine practice for the next generation of internists. Neth J Med. 2015;73(3):100–7.

Pneumothorax of the Newborn

9

Jing Liu, Hai-Ying Cao, and Erich Sorantin

9.1 Pneumothorax

The pleural cavity consists of the parietal pleura and the visceral layer, and it is a gas-free potential enclosed lacuna. After pleural rupture for any reason, the formation of pneumatosis in the thoracic cavity after the air enters the pleura is called pneumothorax, which is a common and critical neonatal illness in clinics and a common cause of death among newborns and preterm infants [1, 2].

9.1.1 Etiology and Pathophysiology

High-risk factors of neonatal pneumothorax include the following:

1. Lung diseases: lung leakage is a common complication of neonatal lung diseases; 27% of lung leakage occurs in infants with hyaline membrane disease, 41% in infants with meconium aspiration syndrome, and 10% in infants with wet lung, pulmonary infection, pulmonary hypoplasia, diaphragmatic hernia, etc.
2. Latrogenic: improper resuscitation, lung iatrogenic fracture, and rib fractures caused by chest compressions.
3. Improper application of ventilator: inspiratory pressure that is too high, end expiratory pressure that is too high, incoordination of respiration, endotracheal intubation position, and suction inducing pulmonary rupture.
4. Spontaneous pneumothorax: for unknown reasons.

The formation of pneumothorax is induced by the following causes: lung tissue bronchi rupture, and air escapes into the pleural cavity; or chest injuries puncture the pleura, the pleural cavity is connected with the outside world, and the outside air enters the pleura. Pneumothorax is the most common form of neonatal pulmonary air leak (including pneumothorax, pneumomediastinum, emphysema, pneumopericardium, and pneumoperitoneum). The heterogeneous alveolar aeration induced by any cause can lead to alveolar rupture, and the gas enters into the pulmonary interstitia to form interstitial emphysema. Interstitial emphysema can directly break into the chest cavity to form pneumothorax, and it can also reach the mediastina to form mediastinal

Electronic Supplementary Material The online version of this chapter (https://doi.org/10.1007/978-94-024-1549-0_9) contains supplementary material, which is available to authorized users.

J. Liu (✉)
Department of Neonatology and NICU,
Beijing Chaoyang District Maternal and Child Health Care Hospital, Beijing, China

H.-Y. Cao
Department of Ultrasound, GE Healthcare, Beijing, China

E. Sorantin
Division of Pediatric Radiology, Department of Radiology, Medical University Graz, Graz, Austria

J. Liu et al. (eds.), *Neonatal Lung Ultrasonography*, https://doi.org/10.1007/978-94-024-1549-0_9

emphysema along the blood vessels, lymphatic vessels, or peribronchial regions. Mediastinal gas can enter the thoracic cavity to form pneumothorax. If the gas enters into the pericardium along large vessels, pneumopericardium is formed; if it enters into the subcutaneous tissues, subcutaneous emphysema is formed; and if it enters into the abdominal cavity, a gas film is formed. It is occasionally seen that the air breaks into the blood capillaries or lymphatic vessels to form aeroembolism. Since the negative pressure in the pleural cavity is neutralized, the wounds and edema site become collapsed. In case of small pneumothorax, in those with lung collapse of less than 30%, the influence on the respiratory and circulatory functions is relatively small, with many obvious clinical symptoms. In case of large pneumothorax, infants can experience dyspnea and cyanosis, the trachea shifts to the healthy side, the percussion of wounded chest presents tympani, and the auscultation indicates that the breath sounds decrease or disappear. Chest X-ray examination might show different degrees of lung collapse and aerothorax sometimes accompanied by a small amount of fluid. After the formation of pneumothorax, the pressure in the pleural cavity increases, and the negative pressures turn into positive pressure, compressing the lungs and blocking the venous blood; therefore, different degrees of pulmonary and heart dysfunctions are produced and are classified into closed pneumothorax, open pneumothorax, and tension pneumothorax.

9.1.1.1 Closed Pneumothorax

Closed pneumothorx, is also known as spontaneous pneumothorax, which is mostly a complication of rib fracture. After the formation of pneumothorax, pneumatosis and compression are seen in the pleural cavity. Visceral pleura rupture is closed so that there is no longer air that continues to be leaked into the pleural cavity.

9.1.1.2 Open Pneumothorax

Open pneumothorax, is also known as communicating pneumothorax, as the chest wall injuries make the outside air go in and out of the pleural cavity freely with respiration, the pressure in the affected pleural cavity is approximately 0. After air exhaust, it is observed that the pressure in the pleural cavity does not decrease. The pathophysiology of open pneumothorax is as follows:

(a) The negative pressure of the pleural cavity disappears; the lungs are compressed to collapse; the pressures at the bilateral pleural cavities are equal, making the bilateral mediastinal shift; and the pulmonary dilation at the healthy side is then limited.
(b) Upon inspiration, the negative pressure at the healthy side of the pleural cavity increases, and the difference with the pressure at the wounded side increases, causing the mediastina to further shift; upon expiration, the difference in the pressures on the bilateral sides of the pleural cavity decreases, the mediastina then shifts back to the wounded side, and this abnormal movement is called mediastinal flutter. Mediastinal flutter can affect venous return, resulting in severe circulatory disorder.
(c) Upon inspiration, the healthy side becomes dilated and inhales the outside air, and the gas with a low oxygen content discharges from the wounded side; upon expiration, some of the gas expired from the healthy side enters the wounded side, and some is discharged through the upper respiratory tract; because the gas with a low oxygen content is exchanged at the two lungs, the anoxia and dyspnea become aggravated.

9.1.1.3 Tension Pneumothorax

Tension pneumothorax, is also known as pressure pneumothorax, the most common reasons is alveolar lacerated wound or bronchial rupture, a flap obstruction is formed at the pleural cleft. Upon inspiration, the open air enters the pleural cavity from the cleft; in respiration, the flap is opened, and the cleft in the pleural cavity returns and is discharged from the respiratory tract. The increasing accumulation of gas in the pleural cavity and the constantly rising pressure form high pressure in the pleural cavity, so the collapse of the injured side of the lung becomes aggravated, the mediastina are pushed to the healthy side under the gradually increased pressure, and the healthy side of the lung is squeezed, resulting in severe respiratory and circulatory disorder. Sometimes, the high-pressure air of the pleural cavity is pushed in the mediastina, spreads to the subcutaneous tissues, and forms subcutaneous emphysema in the neck, face, chest, etc. Air discharge is needed to relieve the symptoms. If gas is sucked until negative pressure is achieved, the positive pressure is not restored quickly, and pleural cavity air discharge equipment should be installed.

9.1.2 Clinical Manifestations

In cases of small pneumothorax, in those with lung collapse of less than 30%, the influence on the respiratory and circulatory functions is relatively small with many obvious clinical symptoms.

In cases of large pneumothorax, the main reasons include the following: the conditions suddenly deteriorate, dyspnea and cyanosis become suddenly worsened, the patient feels listless and inert with low reactions, bilateral breasts are asymmetric, the affected side of the thorax is bulging and full, the respiratory movement becomes weakened with tympani, auscultation indicates that the respiratory sound becomes diminished or disappears, the trachea shifts, the heart rhythm becomes slow, the heart sound is low and distant, and there might be sudden cardiac arrest, decreased blood pressure, and even shock. Obvious collapse and pneumatosis of the pleural cavity are seen on chest X-ray examination, and no markings are visible outside of the pneumothorax line. Mediastinal organs such as the trachea and heart shift to the healthy side of the lungs with the manifestations of decreased diaphragmatic muscle and compression of the healthy side of lungs, and sometimes, a small amount of pleural effusion could be heard. The appearance of a photic zone beside the mediastina suggests mediastinal emphysema. Blood gas analysis shows decreased PaO_2 and increased $PaCO_2$. X-ray examination can identify congenital pulmonary cysts, hernia, and other lung diseases.

9.1.3 Auxiliary Examination

Chest X-ray diagnosis is the most common diagnostic tool for pneumothorax, but its sensitivity and accuracy are not high. It has been reported that pneumothorax in nearly 55% of patients with chest injuries cannot be diagnosed by chest X-ray. CT examination is the gold standard for diagnosis of pneumothorax, but there are some flaws, such as severe radiation injury, the need to transport critically ill patients, and relatively high costs.

9.1.4 Treatment of Pneumothorax

The principle for pneumothorax treatment is to discharge gas properly according to the different types of pneumothorax for the purpose of relieving the respiratory and circulatory disturbances resulting from the aerothorax so that the lung recruitment functions can be recovered as soon as possible and to meanwhile provide active therapies for complications and primary diseases.

1. Gas discharging method: An evaluation is made regarding whether it is necessary to perform gas discharging treatment and what gas discharging method is selected according to the symptoms, signs, X-ray images, and other factors for the judgment of pneumothorax.
2. Closed pneumothorax: For those with small pneumothorax and lung collapse of less than 20–30%, the effect on pulmonary respiration and circulation is not great, and the gas can be self-absorbed in 1–2 weeks without the need for pumping, and dynamic observation is performed. The gas volume is relatively high, gas is pumped once every day or every other day until most of the pulmonary recruitment functions are recovered, and the remaining pneumatosis is absorbed.
3. *Tension pneumothorax*
   (a) Simple approach for air exhaustion: A scalp needle for intravenous infusion is used for puncture and degassing and is connected to a 20–50 ml syringe; the needle is inserted at the second intercostal of the midclavicular line or the fourth to fifth intercostal of the anterior axillary line along the upper margin of ribs, and gas discharge can be seen after the thoracic cavity is entered. Hemostatic forceps are

closely attached to the skin to fix the needle tip until no gas can be discharged. After the needle is pulled out, X-ray radiography is performed to visualize the recruitment. After the needle is pulled out, re-disinfection is performed at the posterior region, which is covered by sterile gauze attached with adhesive tape.

(b) Thoracic cavity closed drainage: (1) The patient is lying in the supine position. (2) The second intercostal at the midclavicular line or the fourth to fifth intercostal at the anterior axillary line serves as the puncture site. (3) Antiseptic facemasks and gloves should be worn to disinfect the skin according to routine procedures. (4) A small incision is made at the upper margin of the ribs at the puncture site after local anesthesia. Cut the skin and subcutaneous tissues, perform blunt dissection of muscles, clamp the transparent catheter with the style with a Venturi forceps (or 8Fr or 10Fr latex catheters), insert the catheter along the incision at the site 1.5–2.0 cm away from the top (45° to the plane), pull out the needles after the pleural cavity is entered (clamp the catheter when it is halfway pulled), and then pull all of them out to prevent the entry of air. Then, propel the needle into the thoracic cavity by 2–3 cm. (5) Perform purse string suture at the incision, fix the catheter, perform disinfection, cover it with sterile gauze, and fix with sticky cloth. Chest X-ray is used to examine the catheter position. (6) Connect the catheter and pneumothorax drainage equipment. (7) After the symptoms disappear, there is no gas suction in the thoracic cavity catheter. Chest X-ray indicates that pneumothorax disappears over 24–48 h. End negative pressure aspiration and clamp the catheter. In cases of no signs of air leakage after 0–12 h, the catheter can be pulled. (8) After pulling out the catheter, suture the incisions, re-disinfect the wound, and cover it with sterile gauze for fixation. (9) If the drainage using this water-sealed bottle cannot heal the pleural crevasse, fluoroscopy indicates that the lungs cannot be recruited persistently, and negative-pressure enclosed drainage equipment is added at the end of the previous drainage. As the aspirator can form injuries induced by excessive negative pressure, the pressure-adjusting bottle can be used to ensure that the negative pressure does not exceed −0.8 to 1.2 kpa (−8 to 12 cmH_2O); if this negative pressure is exceeded, the internal air will enter the pressure-adjusting bottle through the pressure-adjusting catheter; therefore, the aspiration negative pressure imposed on the patient's thoracic cavity is over −8 to 12 cmH_2O. In cases using the closed negative pressure aspiration, it is proper to continuously perform aspiration. If the lungs still cannot recover recruitment function for more than 12 h, the cause should be found. (10) Change the disinfection water-sealed bottles and tubes every day.

4. Pneumothorax occurs with the application of an artificial ventilator during treatment; in cases of mediastinal emphysema, the parameter-adjusting principles are as follows: use a higher frequency such as increased oxygen concentration and a shorter inspiratory time, lower the blood pressure through inspiration and PEEP, and maintain normal blood gas (the water-sealed bottle is connected to the negative-pressure inspiration equipment).
5. Subcutaneous emphysema and concentration of oxygen inside the mediastina facilitate the dissipation of emphysema. Most neonate mediastinal edemas are at the anterior mediastina, which is a potential space between the chest bone and pericardium without important vascular nerves, and the gap becomes widened after pneumatosis and is filled with gas. The puncture is safe and effective, the lateral margins of the chest bones are chosen for puncture and decompression, and good efficacy can be achieved.
6. Emergency treatment of open pneumothorax: first use sterile dressings such as petrolatum gauze cotton pads to seal the wounds, then use

tape or bandages for bandaging and fixation so that the open pneumothorax and closed pneumothorax are connected, and finally, puncture the pleural cavity and suck air for compression and to temporarily relieve dyspnea. Then, perform further treatment.

9.2 Ultrasound Diagnosis of Pneumothorax

9.2.1 Ultrasound Manifestations of Pneumothorax

In recent years, ultrasound has been successfully used to diagnose lung pneumothorax, and ultrasound examination can be used conveniently, more quickly, and more reliably to diagnose pneumothorax. Lung ultrasound is superior to traditional X-ray examination in diagnosing pneumothorax or ruling out pneumothorax [3–6]. Recently, a systemic review and meta-analysis involving 864 cases of adult pneumothorax by Alrajhi et al. [7] showed that the sensitivity and specificity of pneumothorax diagnosis using ultrasound reached 91% and 98.2%, respectively [8]. In examination, priority is given to microconvex transducers, and other transducers such as line array, phase array, or convex array transducers can also be selected. In application of ultrasound for diagnosing pneumothorax, the patient can be in the sitting or supine positions. When in the supine position, pay attention to the anterior chest wall and lateral chest wall, and perform scanning on each intercostal space at the clavicular midline, anterior axillary line, and middle axillary line. During scanning, the transducer might be perpendicular to the ribs and can also be parallel to the intercostal space, and each intercostal space should be scanned for 4–5 breathing cycles. When the patient is in the sitting position, pay attention to scanning the apex of the lungs; in cases of detection of suspicious regions, perform a scan on key regions. The main ultrasound imaging feature of pneumothorax (the sensitivity of the lung point upon diagnosis of pneumothorax is 66%, and the specificity is 100%) includes a clear presence of a lung point, and a lung point is a highly specific sign for diagnosing pneumothorax; M-ultrasound can provide more clear identification of lung points. Disappearance of pneumothorax (the negative predictive value of using lung sliding for pneumothorax is 99.2–100%), disappearance of pleural liens, and no comet tail sign or B-lines, such as the presence of enhanced images, can rule out pneumothorax (the negative predictive value of using comet tail sign or B-lines for pneumothorax is 99.2–100%) and are formed by multiple reflections induced by gas. When the A-lines of pneumothorax patients are present, if lung sliding disappears but the A-line exists, the sensitivity and specificity for the diagnosis of recessive pneumothorax are 95% and 94%. Therefore, in the first examination, first observe the presence of lung sliding; in the case of lung sliding, the presence of pneumothorax is ruled out; if lung sliding is not found, then observe the existence of the comet tail sign; in case of the presence of the comet tail sign, pneumothorax can also be ruled out. If lung sliding and the comet tail sign are not found, we need to consider the possibility of pneumothorax. Further observe whether there might be lung points; if lung points are found, the diagnosis of pneumothorax can be made; if these three signs cannot be observed, the diagnosis of pneumothorax cannot be confirmed. The sensitivity of ultrasound is superior to that of chest X-ray examination, especially in the diagnosis of occult pneumothorax. Lichtenstein et al. carried out retrospective studies on 200 cases of ICU patients, and the ICU physician performed ultrasound scanning with CT as the criterion. When only the disappearance of signs of lung sliding was used as the basis for the diagnosis of pneumothorax, the sensitivity was 100% and the specificity was 78%; when the disappearance of lung sliding and only the detection of A-lines were used as the diagnostic criteria, the sensitivity was 95% and the specificity was 94%. If the signs of lung sliding disappear, the detection of A-lines and the detection of lung points were used, and the sensitivity and specificity were 79% and 100%, respectively.

It can be seen that the use of lung ultrasound to diagnose pneumothorax is mainly based on the following four signs [9, 10]: (1) the presence of lung points, (2) the disappearance of lung sliding, (3) the disappearance of B-lines, and (4) the exist of pleural line and A-lines. The procedures for diagnosing pneumothorax are shown in Fig. 9.1.

9.2.2 Precaution when Using Lung Ultrasound Examination for Diagnosing Pneumothorax

When applying ultrasound for diagnosing pneumothorax, the patient can be in the sitting and supine positions. When the patient is in the supine position, pay attention to check the anterior chest wall and lateral chest wall, and perform scanning on each intercostal space at the clavicular midline, anterior axillary line, and middle axillary line. The transducer can be vertical or parallel to the ribs. When the ultrasound transducer is perpendicular to the ribs for scanning, the acoustic shadows of the ribs to assess signs such as the pleural line and each intercostal space should be scanned for four to five respiratory cycles. When the patient is in the sitting position, pay attention to scanning the apex of the lungs; in cases of detection of suspicious regions, perform scanning on key regions. In the examination, the patient's medical history and physical signs are combined for comprehensive consideration. First, observe the presence of lung sliding. In cases of lung sliding, the presence of pneumothorax is ruled out; if lung sliding is not found, then observe the existence of the comet tail sign. In cases of the presence of the comet tail sign, pneumothorax can also be ruled out. If lung sliding and the comet tail sign are not found, we need to consider the possibility of pneumothorax. Further observe whether there might be lung points; if lung points are found, the diagnosis of pneumothorax can be made. If these three signs cannot be observed, the diagnosis of pneumothorax cannot be confirmed.

9.2.3 Experience from Our Team

According to our experience in this field, the main sonographic signs of neonatal pneumothorax include the disappearance of lung sliding via real-time ultrasound, no B-lines or lung consolidation, and the existence of the pleural line and A-line; in addition, mild-moderate patients also present lung points [7]. Regarding these signs, several key points emerge [7]. (1) In our population, the disappearance of lung sliding under real-time ultrasound is the most valuable ultrasonic sign. If lung sliding disappears and B-line or lung consolidation is not observed, the presence of pneumothorax is essentially confirmed. (2) Patients with pneumothoraxes do not present lung sliding, B-line, or lung consolidation. If any one of these signs is present, pneumothorax can be excluded. However, because the majority of normal neonates do not have the B-line, its absence does not necessarily indicate pneumothorax. Therefore, this finding should be combined with other signs. In addition, lung sliding also disappears during severe lung consolidation (such as large areas of atelectasis) [11]. Therefore, for neonatal patients with disappearance of lung sliding to be considered to have pneumothorax, lung consolidation should be excluded. Nonetheless, the presence of lung sliding can definitely exclude pneumothorax [12]. (3) All of the patients with pneumothoraces had existing pleural lines and A-lines. The sensitivity and specificity of the diagnosis of pneumothorax using the disappearance of lung sliding and the presence of the pleural line and A-line were both 100%. (4) The lung point is not the most sensitive sign for pneumothorax diagnosis. Particularly in severe pneumothorax, the areas below the probe are all air; therefore, the lung point is not present. However, this feature is the most specific sign for pneumothorax diagnosis. If this sign is discovered, the specificity of diagnosis of mild-moderate pneumothorax is 100%, and the presence of (mild-moderate) pneumothorax can be confirmed [13]. Because neonates have faster respiratory rates under normal conditions, the respiratory rates of pediatric patients will significantly increase after the development of pneumothorax. Because their respiratory rates are very fast, the cutoff point, i.e., the lung point, between normal and abnormal cannot be clearly displayed in a shorter time under the probe. Therefore, when pneumothorax is suspected, lung sliding should first be evaluated under real-time ultrasound. If a lack of lung sliding and lung point is identified, then pneumothorax can be diagnosed. Therefore, the disappearance of lung sliding under real-time ultrasound is the most important ultrasonic feature and is the key for the diagnosis of pneumothorax using ultrasound.

Our study also found that both the positive and negative predictive values of the disappearance of lung sliding and the existence of pleural lines and A-lines in diagnosing pneumothorax by ultrasound were 100% [7]. The presence of the lung points indicates a mild to moderate pneumothorax; otherwise, the pneumothorax would be severe. Therefore, these three signs, the disappearance of lung sliding, existence of the pleural line and A-line, and the lung point, are the decisive factors for the diagnosis of or exclusion of pneumothorax.

M-mode ultrasound is also usually used for pneumothorax diagnosis. Under M-type ultrasound, the "seashore" sign of normal lung tissues is replaced by the "parallel sign" formed by intrathoracic gas [13]. Then, the lung point or parallel sign t found by M-mode ultrasound would further confirm the existence of pneumothorax. The disappearance of lung sliding under B-type ultrasound is the first and most important step in the diagnosis of pneumothorax using ultrasound [7].

Although the diagnosis of lung diseases using ultrasound is simple overall, the diagnosis of neonatal pneumothorax using ultrasound is relatively difficult; skill in this technique is also the most difficult to achieve and is significantly different in neonates compared to adults. The main reason for the difficulty is that after the development of pneumothorax, the neonates' difficulty breathing further significantly increased on the basis of their original lung diseases; therefore, the lung point is difficult to identify when the respiratory rate is very fast. Therefore, when using ultrasound for the diagnosis of neonatal pneumothorax, proper training and certain levels of experience are required [14]. Based on our experiences and observations, for neonatal patients with suspected pneumothorax in the clinic, the presence of lung sliding is the first sign observed via real-time ultrasound (Fig. 9.1). (1) If lung sliding is present, then pneumothorax is essentially excluded. (2) If lung sliding disappears, (a) the lung point and pleural line and A-line are searched—if they are present, pneumothorax can be diagnosed; (b) the B-line and atelectasis should be checked. If no B-line is detected, the presence of pneumothorax can be essentially confirmed. If a B line is present, pneumothorax can be excluded. (3) If necessary, the M-mode ultrasound can also be used to find the lung point or parallel sign, which confirms the pneumothorax (Figs. 9.2, 9.3, 9.4, 9.5, 9.6, and 9.8).

We stated that all the pictures or ultrasound images included in the chapter were taken from

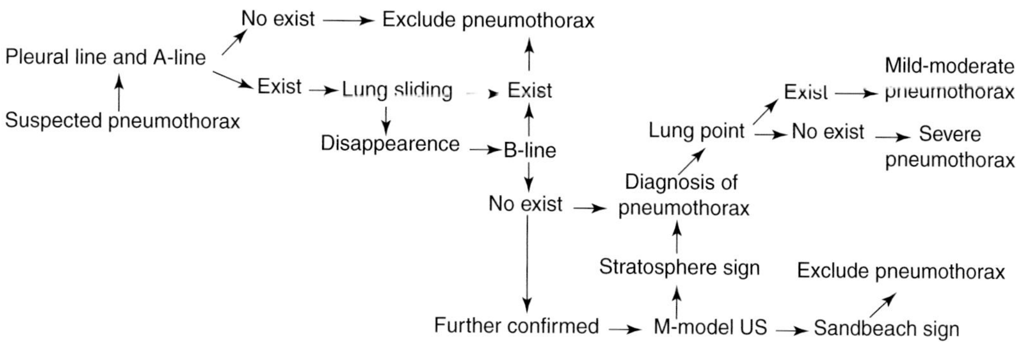

Fig. 9.1 The flowchart for neonatal pneumothorax

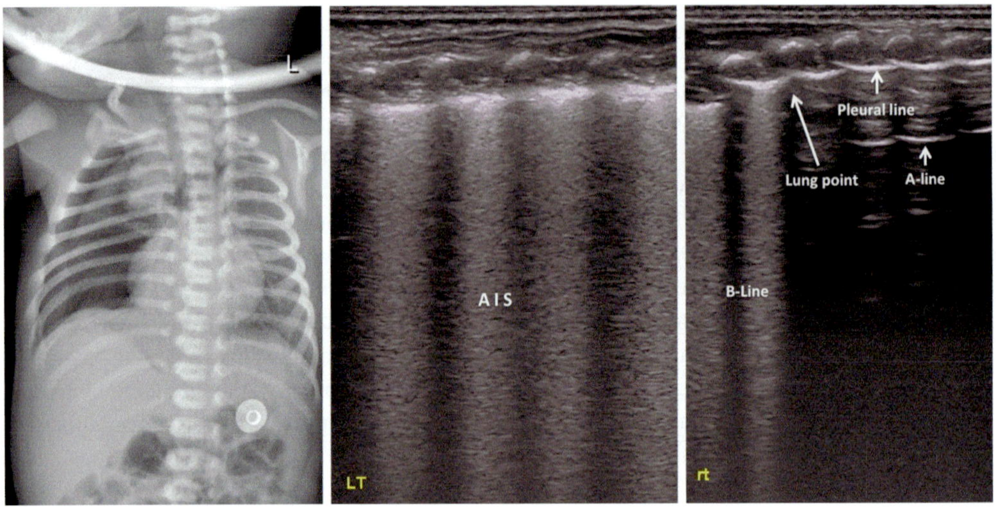

Fig. 9.2 Ultrasonic manifestation of mild-moderate pneumothorax in a transient tachypnea of the newborn (TTN) patient. The gestational age (GA) and birth weight of this baby, who was admitted to our NICU because of breathing difficulties for 4 h with a diagnosis of TTN, were 38 weeks and 2550 g, respectively. The lung ultrasound showed an abnormal pleural line, adenocarcinoma in situ (AIS), and disappearing A-lines in the left lung, whereas the right lung shows the lung point, that is, the transition from the B-line area (*left side*) to a hypoechoic area with horizontal reverberations of the parietal pleura in the right side. Under real-time ultrasound, the lung sliding was occurring in the B-line area, while it was disappearing in the A-line area (also see Video 9.1)

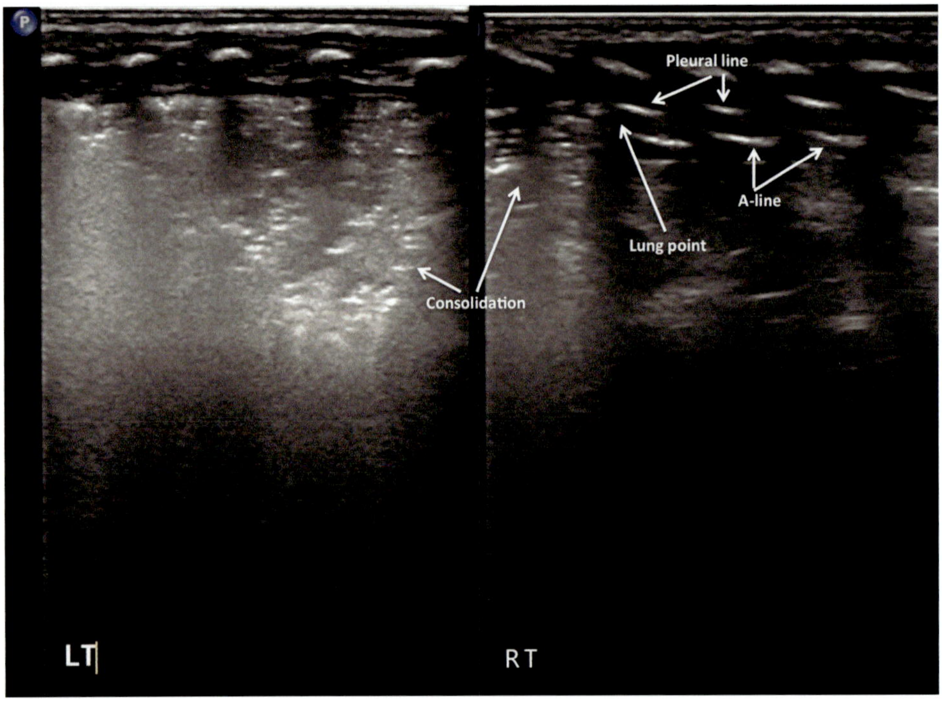

Fig. 9.3 Ultrasonic manifestation of mild-moderate pneumothorax in a respiratory distress (RDS) patient. The infant had a GA of 37^{+6} weeks and was delivered by cesarean section with a birth weight of 2850 g. The infant was admitted to our NICU because of severe dyspnea for 32 h. The lung ultrasound showed a large area of lung consolidation with significant air bronchograms in the left lung and a small area of lung consolidation with air bronchograms in the left side of the right lung; there were clear pleural lines and A-lines on the right side of the right lung. Under real-time ultrasound, lung sliding was occurring in the consolidation area, while it was disappearing in the A-line area (also see Video 9.2)

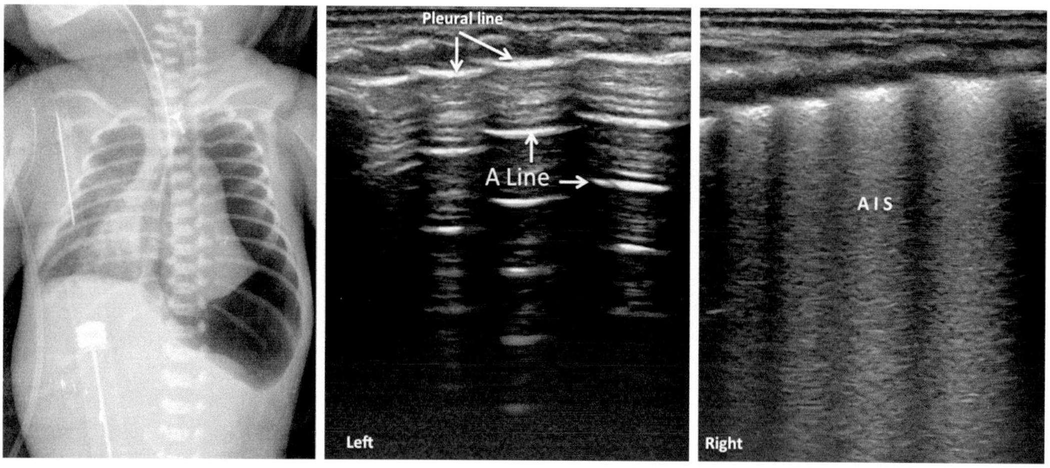

Fig. 9.4 Ultrasonic manifestation of severe pneumothorax in a TTN patient. The GA of the infant was 32 weeks, and the birth weight was 2400 g; the infant was admitted to our NICU due to breathing difficulties for 4 h. The chest X-ray showed severe pneumothorax in the left lung. The lung ultrasound showed AIS in the right lung and pleural line as well as A-lines in the left lung, whereas no lung point was found in the left lung. Under real-time ultrasound, the lung sliding was disappearing in the whole right lung field, while it was appearing in the left lung (also see Videos 9.3 and 9.4)

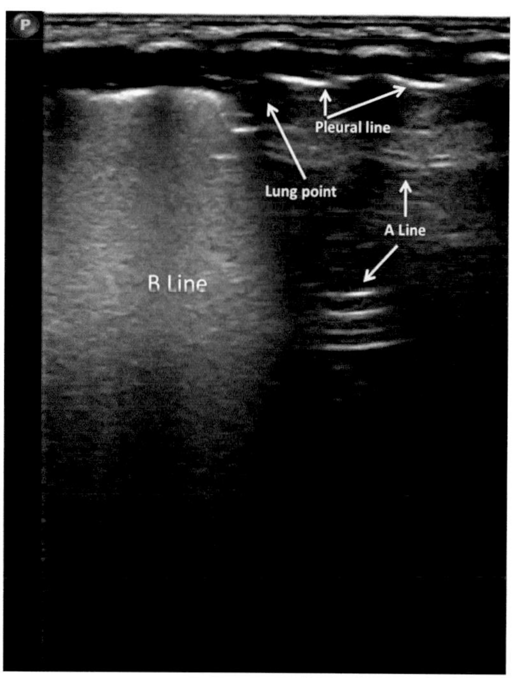

Fig. 9.5 Ultrasonic manifestation of pneumothorax. Ultrasound lung scan in B mode showing the lung point, that is, the transition from the B-line area (*left side*) to a hypoechoic area (*right side*). Under real-time ultrasound, lung sliding is occurring in the B-line area, while it is disappearing on the right side of the same picture; the point of demarcation between the consolidation and the right side of the same picture was the lung point (Video 9.5)

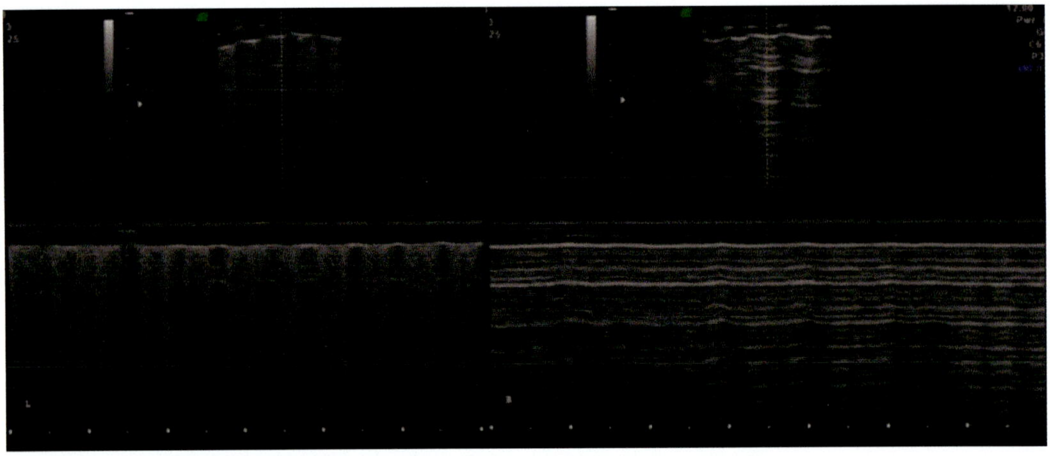

Fig. 9.6 Severe pneumothorax under M-model ultrasound. Under M-model ultrasound, the left lung showed the beach sign, while the right lung presented the stratosphere sign (also known as barcode sign), which confirmed the severe pneumothorax in the right thorax

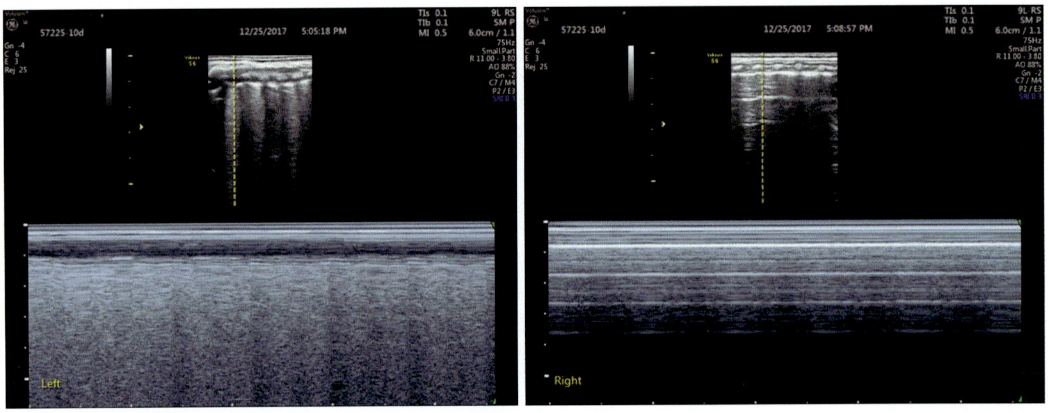

Fig. 9.7 Severe pneumothorax. Severe pneumothorax in the right thorax. M-model ultrasound showed that beach sign in the left lung, while the stratosphere sign in the right lung

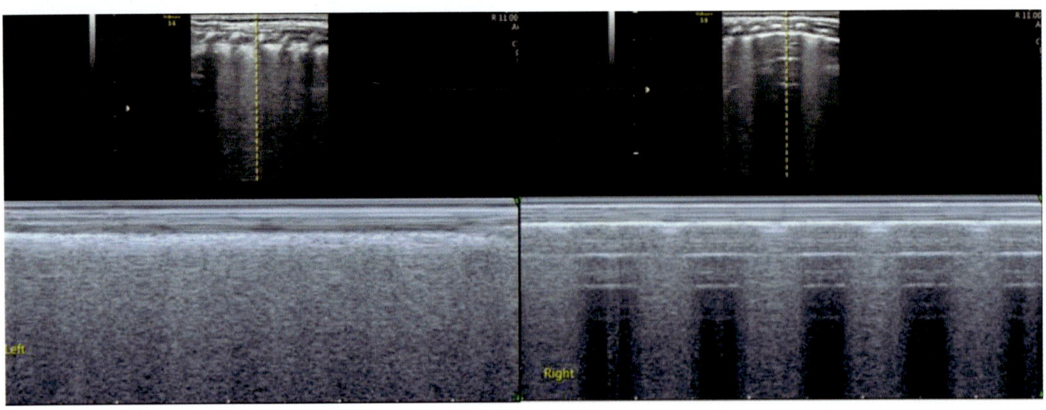

Fig. 9.8 Mild pneumothorax under M-model ultrasound. Under M-model ultrasound, the left lung showed beach signs, while the right lung presented the lung point (the point that appears opposite of the beach sign and the stratosphere sign), which confirmed the mild pneumothorax in the right thorax

the Army General Hospital of the Chinese PLA and Beijing Chaoyang District Maternal and Child Healthcare Hospital; the related studies were approved by both the committee of the Army General Hospital and Chaoyang District Maternal and Child Healthcare Hospital.

9.2.4 Limitations of Using Ultrasound to Diagnose Pneumothorax

There are some limitations of using ultrasound to diagnose pneumothorax. The results of ultrasound examination are greatly subject to the skill level of the examinees, and the judgment on the ultrasound images directly affects the accuracy of the results. For example, under normal conditions and in the case of pneumothorax, vertical hyperechoic strips that stem from the pleural lines can be seen. What is different from B-lines is that these echo strips will become attenuated and disappear (cannot reach the edge of screen) after a certain distance, cannot cover A-lines, cannot move with respiration, and need to be differentiated with comet tail signs. In cases of emphysema of the periphery of the lungs, the high echo strips perpendicularly originate from the superficial surface tissues and reach the edge of screen. At this time, the shadows of the pleural lines and ribs are invisible and need to be differentiated with B-lines. A-lines can be seen in normal lungs, some diseases, and pneumothorax. When ultrasound examination is applied, it is necessary to reasonably select the imaging criteria, and further studies are needed for the more accurate and reliable ultrasound signs. The dressings for bandaging the chest wall skin injuries and local wounds will limit the use of ultrasound examination, and subcutaneous emphysema might affect the examination results.

References

1. Duong HH, Mirea L, Shah PS, et al. Pneumothorax in neonates: trends, predictors and outcomes. J Neonatal Perinatal Med. 2014;7:29–38.
2. Bhatia R, Davis PG, Doyle LW, et al. Identification of pneumothorax in very preterm infants. J Pediatr. 2011;159:115–20.
3. Volpicelli G. Sonographic diagnosis of pneumothorax. Intensive Care Med. 2011;37:224–32.
4. Alrajab S, Youssef AM, Akkus NI, Caldito G. Pleural ultrasonography versus chest radiography for the diagnosis of pneumothorax: review of the literature and meta-analysis. Crit Care. 2013;17:R208.
5. Raimondi F, Fanjul JR, Aversa S, et al. Lung ultrasound for diagnosing pneumothorax in the critically ill neonate. J Pediatr. 2016;175(8):74–78.e1.
6. Alrajhi K, Woo MY, Vaillancourt C. Test characteristics of ultrasonography for the detection of pneumothorax: a systematic review and meta-analysis. Chest. 2012;141:703–8.
7. Liu J, Chi JH, Ren XL, et al. Lung ultrasonography to diagnose pneumothorax of the newborn. Am J Emerg Med. 2017;35(9):1298–302.
8. Berlet T, Fehr T, Merz TM. Current practice of lung ultrasonography (LUS) in the diagnosis of pneumothorax: a survey of physician monographers in Germany. Crit Ultrasound J. 2014;6:16.
9. Volpicelli G, Elbarbary M, Blaivas M, et al. International evidence-based recommendations for point-of-care lung ultrasound. Intensive Care Med. 2012;38(4):577–91.
10. Liu J, Feng X, Hu CB, et al. Guideline on lung ultrasound to diagnose pulmonary diseases in newborn infants. Chin J Appl Clin Pediatr. 2018;33(14):1057–64.
11. Liu J, Chen SW, Liu F, et al. The diagnosis of neonatal pulmonary atelectasis using lung ultrasonography. Chest. 2015;147(4):1013–9.
12. Lichtenstein DA, Menu YA. Bedside ultrasound sign ruling out pneumothorax in the critically ill: lung sliding. Chest. 1995;108(5):1345–8.
13. Lichtenstein D, Mezie're G, Biderman P, et al. The 'lung point': an ultrasound sign specific to pneumothorax. Intensive Care Med. 2000;26(11):1434–40.
14. Krishnan S, Kuhl T, Ahmed W, Togashi K, Ueda K. Efficacy of an online education program for ultrasound diagnosis of pneumothorax. Anesthesiology. 2013;118:715–21.

Beyond Diagnosis

10

Jing Liu

10.1 Lung Ultrasound Monitoring to Guide Ventilator Withdrawal

Neonatal respiratory failure due to various reasons is the main cause of neonatal hospitalization, and mechanical ventilation is indispensable for respiratory failure rescue therapy and treatment success. Mechanical ventilation therapy can improve lung ventilation and gas exchange, correct hypoxemia and hypercapnia, improve hypoxia, and buy valuable time for the treatment of the primary diseases causing respiratory failure. Currently, frequently used ventilation modes include conventional mechanical ventilation (CMV) and high-frequency ventilation (HFV).

10.1.1 Indications for Neonatal Mechanical Ventilation

Dyspnea due to various causes is an indication for neonatal mechanical ventilation. The relative indications for mechanical ventilation in newborns include the following: (1) frequent apnea and drug intervention ineffectiveness; (2) a sharp deterioration in arterial blood gas analysis, making mechanical ventilation difficult to avoid; (3) severe dyspnea (the early application of mechanical ventilation can relieve the work of breathing); and (4) a requirement for exogenous pulmonary surfactant. The absolute indications include the following: (1) long-term apnea; (2) $FiO_2 > 0.6$–0.7 and $PaO_2 < 50$–60 mmHg (except in cyanotic heart disease); (3) $PaCO_2 > 60$ mmHg, pH <7.20–7.25; and (4) generalized anesthesia.

The indications for HFV include (1) heterogeneous lung diseases, such as meconium aspiration syndrome, pneumothorax, interstitial emphysema, congenital diaphragmatic hernia, pulmonary hemorrhage, pneumonia, congenital diaphragmatic hernia, or induced pulmonary hypoplasia; (2) serious heterogeneous lung disease, such as RDS or pulmonary edema; and (3) other diseases, such as persistent pulmonary hypertension, severe scleroderma, necrotizing enterocolitis, severe abdominal distension, or thoracic deformities. Traditionally or habitually, the majority of physicians often use high-frequency ventilation when the efficacy of normal frequency mechanical ventilation is poor or ineffective, and an indication for HFV is when normal ventilation cannot be maintained with a PIP $\geq$ 25 cmH_2O, MAP $\geq$12 cmH_2O, and $FiO_2 \geq 60\%$. Wunsch et al. conducted an evidence-based medicine analysis of the literature related to the abovementioned topics by searching well-

Electronic Supplementary Material The online version of this chapter (https://doi.org/10.1007/978-94-024-1549-0_10) contains supplementary material, which is available to authorized users.

J. Liu
Department of Neonatology and NICU,
Beijing Chaoyang District Maternal and Child Healthcare Hospital, Beijing, China

J. Liu et al. (eds.), *Neonatal Lung Ultrasonography*, https://doi.org/10.1007/978-94-024-1549-0_10

known databases, such as the fourth version of the Cochrane Library (2002), MEDLINE (1966–2002.10), EMBASE (1980–2002.11), World Wide Web and Web of Science (1988–2002), and EBM, at different time points, and the results showed that there was no evidence suggesting that high-frequency ventilation reduced the mortality and long-term morbidity of acute lung injury and acute respiratory distress syndrome. Thus, high-frequency ventilation should not be used as an alternative to normal-frequency ventilation, and an appropriate ventilation mode should be selected based on the patient's condition and individual experience.

10.1.2 Ultrasound Monitoring to Guide the Withdrawal of Mechanical Ventilation

Clinicians are more familiar with the conditions of respirator withdrawal, which mainly include the following:

1. The causes that led to respiratory failure have been relieved or are being relieved; in premature infants with RDS, relief of these causes may include increases in PS secretions, control of pulmonary infections, correction of shock, improvement in central respiratory failure, and repair of diaphragmatic hernias.
2. The patient's systemic conditions have improved; the general conditions have improved; the mental reactions are fair; the internal environment is normal; any anemia is corrected; and the nutritional status is good.
3. The airway is smooth, the cough reflex is complete, the respiratory muscle strength recovery is good, spontaneous breathing is relatively strong, and function of the respiratory center is normal.
4. Circulation is stable; the patient has stopped taking intravenous vasopressors or cardiac tonics, and no serious arrhythmia has occurred.
5. No muscle relaxants have been used within 12 h.
6. No obvious abdominal distension is present because abdominal distension may cause diaphragmatic elevation and affect the expansion of the thorax, resulting in an increase in respiratory work and failure of machine withdrawal. Although there is no uniform standard for respirator withdrawal, it is generally believed that if the $FiO_2 < 0.4$, RR <15 times/min, PIP <15 cmH_2O, PEEP <4 cmH_2O, and the arterial blood gas analysis is normal, respirator withdrawal can be considered.

However, experience tells us that even if infants meet the abovementioned conditions and standards, when the machine is withdrawn when $FiO_2 = 0.21$, their spontaneous breathing is good, arterial blood gas is normal, and no abnormal findings are observed on a recheck chest X-ray examination, a few infants still need treatment again, and a minority of patients still need to resume respirator support for a single treatment or for multiple additional treatments. By means of lung ultrasound, occult and focal atelectasis can be detected in these infants; when these infants undergo endotracheal lavage and recover from atelectasis, the respirator can be withdrawn smoothly. We performed lung ultrasound examinations on 20 infants who experienced difficulty in ventilator withdrawal, and abnormalities were found in 17 patients. Among them, eight patients experienced focal and recessive atelectasis, five experienced pneumonedema, and four experienced atelectasis accompanied by pneumonedema. It is evident that occult, focal atelectasis and pneumonedema are important causes of difficulty in respirator withdrawal. Lung ultrasound can easily identify the underlying lesions; thus, the original "respirator withdrawal indications" are unreliable, and respirator withdrawal with ultrasound guidance is safer.

According to our experience, neonatal ventilator withdrawal with ultrasound monitoring can follow these rules:

1. In cases of pulmonary disease in which the main feature is lung consolidation, when the

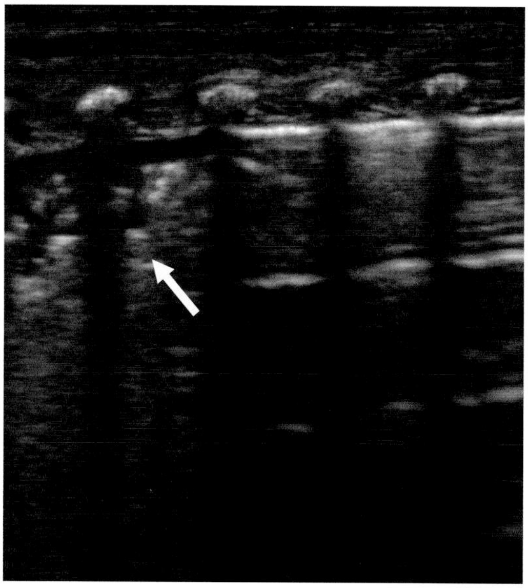

Fig. 10.1 Recessive atelectasis of an infant with difficulty in ventilator withdrawal. The baby was G_2P_1 with gestational age of 38+4 weeks, with respiratory therapy due to MAS. After the clinical symptoms resolved, blood gas analysis and ventilator parameters reached the traditional indications for respirator withdrawal, and the respirator was withdrawn. However, after the respirator was withdrawn, the patient still experienced dyspnea, and a recheck chest X-ray showed no obvious abnormalities. A lung ultrasound shows no abnormalities in the left lower lung field, but focal lung consolidation is present in two intercostal spaces in the upper lung field accompanied by air bronchograms (*arrow*), suggesting the presence of focal occult atelectasis, which is the reason for the difficulty in withdrawing the respirator

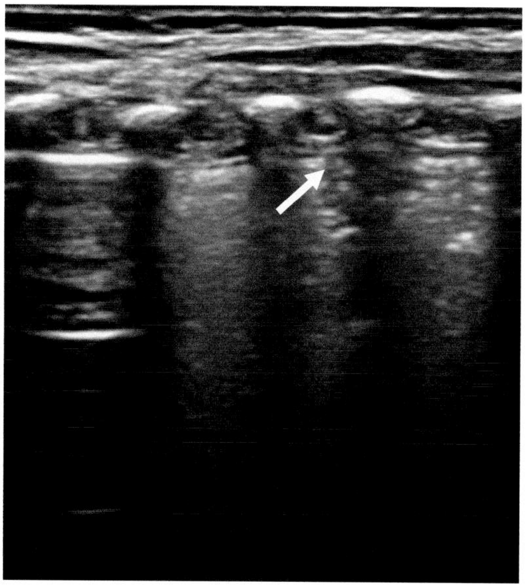

Fig. 10.2 Difficulty in ventilator withdrawal. Gestational age of 37^{+6} weeks. The patient underwent respirator treatment due to RDS; 12 days thereafter, the patient met the criteria for respirator withdrawal, and the respirator was withdrawn. However, soon after respirator withdrawal, the patient experienced dyspnea and respirator treatment was resumed. A lung ultrasound shows that the right upper lung field is normal, and pleural lines and A-lines are clearly visible; the middle lung field shows AIS; and lung consolidation is still present in two intercostal spaces accompanied by air bronchograms (*arrow*) in the lower lung field, suggesting that this side of the lung has not completely returned to normal, which is the reason that the patient needed continued respiratory support

ultrasound examination shows disappearance of the consolidation, when AIS is the main ultrasonographic appearance, withdrawal of the machine can be considered.

2. In cases of pulmonary disease in which the main feature is severe edema (ultrasound images showing a dense B-line and/or white lung, e.g., severe TTN), when the ultrasound examination shows that the edema has been absorbed (mild AIS is the main appearance on the ultrasound images), withdrawal of the machine can be considered.
3. In cases of any kind of lung disease, when the B-line area < 50% of all the lung fields, the ventilator can be safely removed (Figs. 10.1, 10.2, and 10.3).

10.2 Differentiating the Reasons for Long-Term Oxygen Dependence in Premature Infants

Oxygen dependence is a clinically common respiratory system problem in premature infants, especially in smaller premature infants at a gestational age of <32 weeks. In cases in which the demand for oxygen lasts for over 28 days, this is diagnosed as chronic lung disease (CLD) of the newborn or bronchopulmonary dysplasia (BPD). The lower the gestational age as well as the lower the birth weight, the higher the incidence rate of these diseases. Usually, due to immature lung

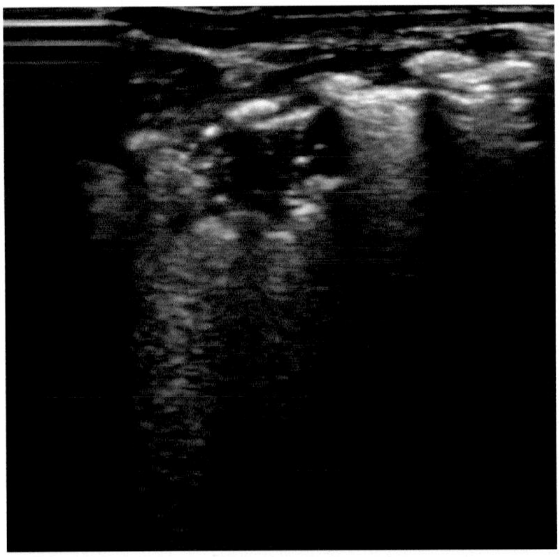

Fig. 10.3 Difficulty in ventilator withdrawal. Gestational age of 27+1weeks, birth weight of 825 g. Mechanical ventilation therapy was provided due to RDS after birth, and 1 week thereafter, the patient met the criteria for respirator withdrawal. However, the patient's dyspnea was still obvious after the respirator was withdrawn. A lung ultrasound shows lung consolidation at less than two intercostal spaces in the middle lung field accompanied by air bronchograms (air), suggesting the presence of focal atelectasis

development in premature infants, acute lung injuries induced by positive pressure ventilation and/or inhalation of high concentrations of oxygen due to treatment of diseases, such as RDS, pneumonia, and MAS, can lead to chronic lung injury and pulmonary function abnormalities and result in the patient's need for auxiliary oxygen. As the survival rate of premature infants increases, the BPD incidence rate displays a year-to-year rising trend, and the quality of life of premature infants is seriously affected.

10.2.1 Clinical Knowledge on BPD

Early in 1967, BPD was first reported and named by Northway et al.; this is considered classic BPD. The main features are as follows: (1) premature infant of a high gestational age and a relatively large birth weight, (2) primary lung disease of severe RDS, (3) history of long-term treatment with 100% oxygen and mechanical ventilation at a high peak inspiratory pressure, (4) continuous oxygen dependence for more than 28 days, and (5) characteristic chest X-ray changes. In recent years, the incidence of classic and severe BPD has been significantly reduced and replaced by a mild form of BPD. In June 2000, the US National Institute of Child Health and Human Development; National Heart, Lung, and Blood Institute; and some other disease commissions jointly organized BPD-themed seminars and reached a consensus at these meetings about using BPD to replace CLD to distinguish it from other chronic lung diseases that occur in infancy; a new definition of BPD was also formulated. According to this definition, for any newborn, as long as the oxygen-dependency duration (>21%) is over 28 days, the diagnosis of BPD can be made. For those of a gestational age <32 weeks, BPD is classified into three types according to the degrees of oxygen dependence at the corrected gestational age of 36 weeks or at discharge: (1) mild with no need to use oxygen, (2) moderate with a requirement for oxygen but an $FiO_2 < 0.3$, and (3) severe with a requirement for oxygen and an $FiO_2 \geq 0.3$ or the need for mechanical ventilation. In cases in which the gestational age $\geq$ 32 weeks, the disease is classified as mild, moderate, or severe according to the oxygen dependence at 56 days after birth or at discharge, and the criteria are the same as previously described. Lung X-ray manifestations do not serve as evidence for the evaluation of disease severity.

However, since 2000, people's perceptions of BPD have not undergone further change, although more than 10 years have passed. Based on our experience and knowledge of BPD, BPD should be defined as a simple pulmonary developmental disorder or dysplasia of newborns that is induced by the combined effects of multiple factors. It can be concomitantly present with other diseases such as lung infections. However, if the oxygen dependence is only due to lung infections, pneumonedema from severe arterial duct patency, or other reasons, the diagnosis is still BPD, which is bound to lead to the expansion of this diagnosis, resulting in a series of medical, nursing, and even ethical problems. Experts report that nearly 50% of BPD patients have a TORCH infection; but do these so-called BPD patients suffer from true BPD, combined BPD and TORCH infection, or a simple TORCH infection instead of BPD? In the last situation, it is clearly inappropriate to diagnose BPD. We also find in clinical practice that, for some patients who are originally highly oxygen dependent, oxygen dependence disappears when lung inflammation is cured; in cases in which ligation of a serious patent atrial duct is performed, the respirator and oxygen dependence resolves.

10.2.2 Use of Lung Ultrasound for Differentiating Oxygen-Dependent Disease States

We have conducted lung ultrasound examinations on 50 BPD patients according to the traditional diagnostic criteria [1]. The results showed that a fairly large number of them did not really suffer from BPD, while others did not have BPD alone (which meaning that they had BPD coexisted with other lung diseases). Therefore, we believe that the long-term oxygen dependence (LTOD) among these infants may have been caused by other pathological changes; thus, it is unreasonable to diagnose BPD in these patients.

Among the 50 patients, there were 9 cases of atelectasis (Fig. 10.4) (4 involving BPD coexisting with atelectasis), 4 cases of pneumonia (Fig. 10.5) (2 involving BPD), 2 patients with severe lung edema, and 3 patients with lung edema accompanied by lung consolidation, which indicated that 36% (18/50) of LTOD patients either did not really have BPD or did not have BPD alone. After endotracheal lavage or pulmonary physical treatment, the infants got significant improvements or complete resolution of respiratory symptoms. Many of these lung diseases are not easily detected by chest X-ray test, while chest CT was not utilized also, and existing lung conditions necessitated the use of LTOD for these infants, finally leading to BPD. We named such kind of BPD as iatrogenic BPD. Thus, it is necessary to revise the diagnostic criteria of BPD and to continue studying and utilizing bedside lung ultrasound as an additional diagnostic tool, as this modality has not been adopted universally [1].

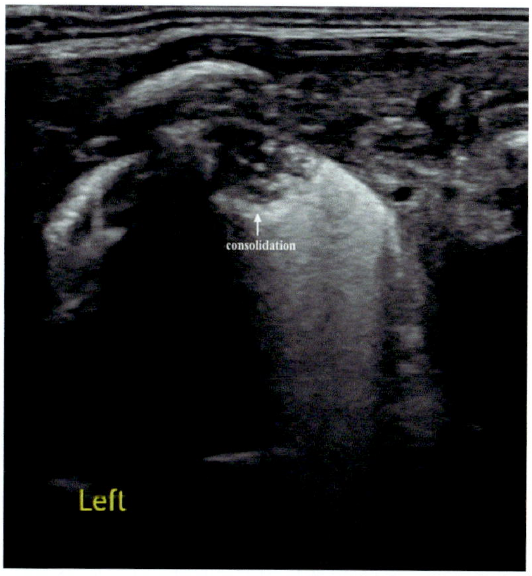

Fig. 10.4 Occult atelectasis. Gestational age of 27^{+3} weeks with birth weight of 975 g. The patient was admitted to the hospital because of RDS and was given mechanical ventilation that lasted for 28 days. Until more than 80 days after birth who still needed to oxygen inhalation and was diagnosed as BPD. Lung ultrasound at 81 days after birth showed lung consolidation with bronchograms within one to two intercostals in the left upper lung field suggesting existing atelectasis, but chest X-ray showed no abnormalities, and the diagnosis was "occult" atelectasis

10.3 Differentiation Between the Thymus and Atelectasis

Generally, the diagnosis of pulmonary atelectasis mainly relies on chest X-rays (Figs. 10.6, 10.7, 10.8, and 10.9); however, in some conditions, a large thymus is frequently misdiagnosed as pulmonary atelectasis by X-ray. However, lung ultrasound can easily distinguish between the thymus and atelectasis [2]. The following are some cases.

Case I: The patient was female, G_2P_2, with a gestational age of 35^{+3} weeks, delivered by cesarean birth, and had no asphyxia at birth. She was admitted to the hospital 10 days after birth because of "difficulty breathing for 10 hours." The patient was admitted to the hospital again 2 months after birth (corrected gestational age, 43 weeks) because of "coughing for 4 days." After admission, she was diagnosed with "neo-

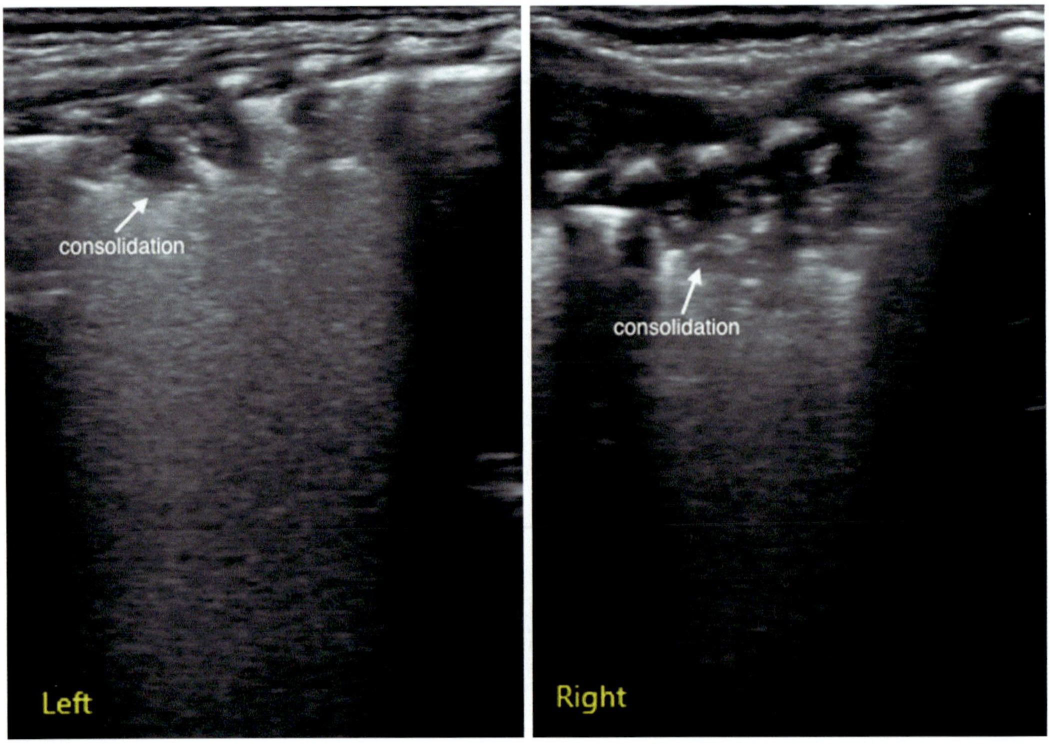

Fig. 10.5 Pneumonia-like findings by lung ultrasound. Gestational age of 28 $^{+5}$ weeks, vaginal delivery with birth weight of 1080 g. The patient was admitted due to extremely premature birth as well as RDS. The respirator was withdrawn 28 days after the initiation of mechanical ventilation. However, after respirator withdrawal, the patient still experienced obvious dyspnea and needed to use nCPAP support and oxygen dependence until 42 days after birth. Lung ultrasound showed significant lung consolidation with bronchograms within bilateral lung fields; the edges of consolidation areas are irregular suggesting the presence of pneumonia of both sides of the lungs

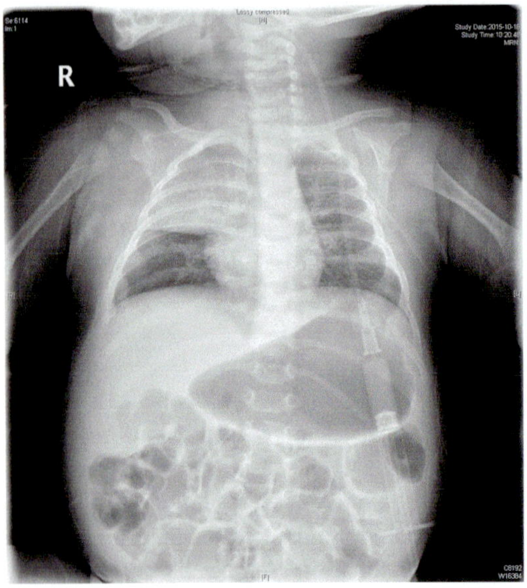

Fig. 10.6 Chest X-ray revealed atelectasis in the right upper lung

natal pneumonia" based on her medical history, physical examination, and lab tests. Twelve days later, the clinical symptoms completely resolved, and lab tests were normal; thus, antibiotic treatment was discontinued, and the patient was ready to be discharged. However, a chest X-ray revealed large, patchy, hyperdensity shadows with clear edges in the right upper lung field, and the patient was suspected of having "right upper lung atelectasis" (Fig. 10.6). However, the patient's general conditions were good, with no signs of difficulty breathing, and a physical examination also revealed no abnormal signs in the lungs. A lung ultrasound (scanned from the patient's back) revealed normal echoes from the lungs, with clear pleural lines and A lines, smooth and regular pleural lines with no thickening or blurring, and no interstitial lung syndrome, consolidation, or air bronchograms; thus, the

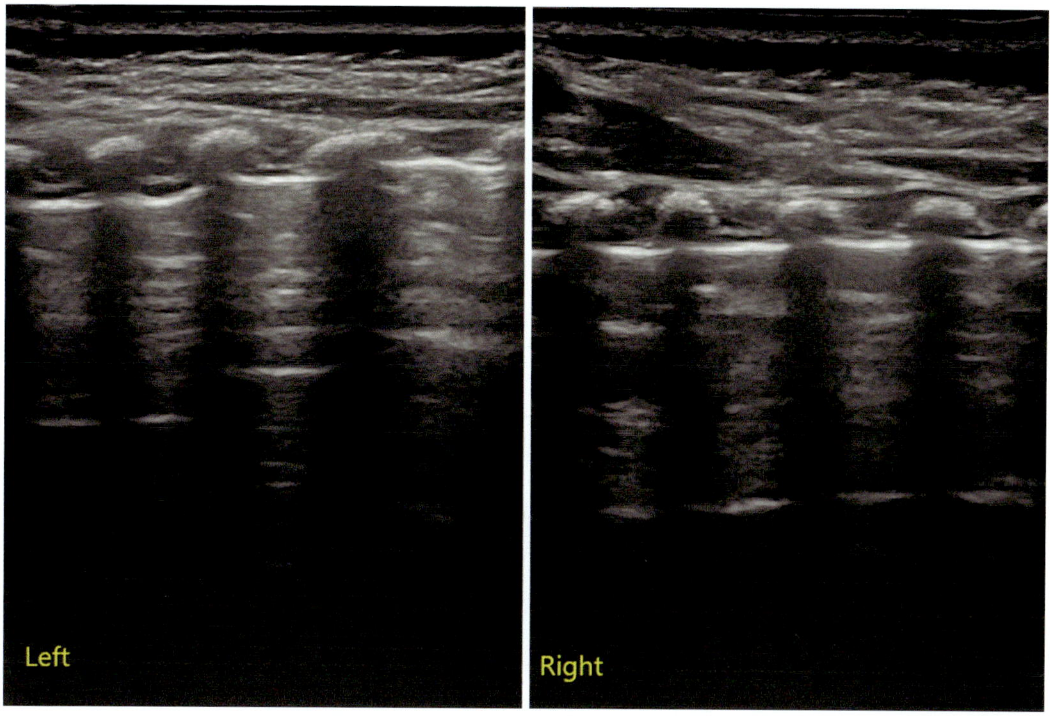

Fig. 10.7 A lung ultrasound (scanned from the patient's back) was normal

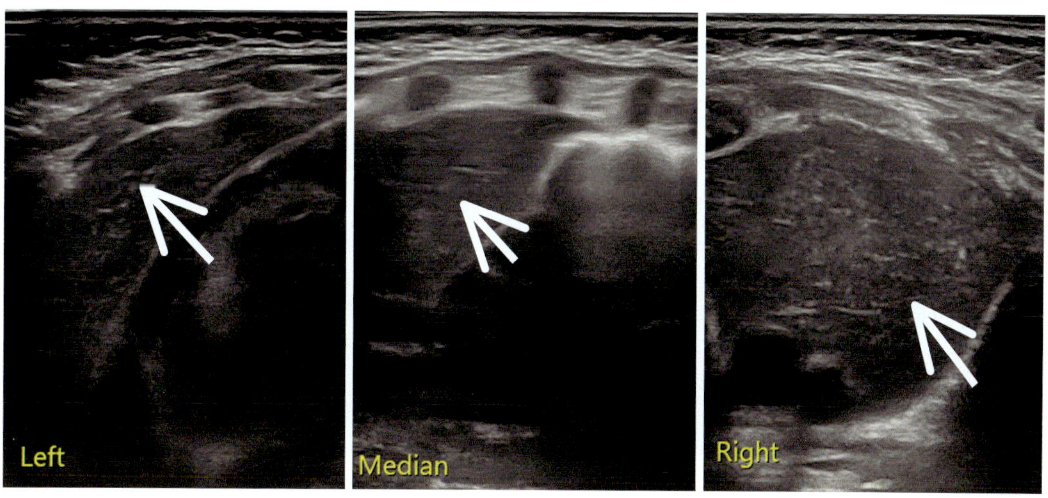

Fig. 10.8 A lung ultrasound (scanned from the patient's front) suggested that the "atelectasis" seen on the previous chest X-ray was the thymus (*arrow*), which was also confirmed by chest CT (Fig. 10.9)

lung ultrasound was normal (Fig. 10.7). A lung ultrasound (scanned from the patient's front) revealed an approximate lumpy parenchymal echo area in the upper chest, with uniform, fine internal echoes and a clear, intact capsule. The mass was primarily located in the right upper chest, with a small portion extending to the mediastinum and the left chest, which was suggestive of the thymus (Fig. 10.8). To further confirm the diagnosis, the patient underwent a lung CT scan, which confirmed that the mediastinal and right upper mediastinal parenchymal echoes detected by the lung ultrasound were from the thymus (Fig. 10.9).

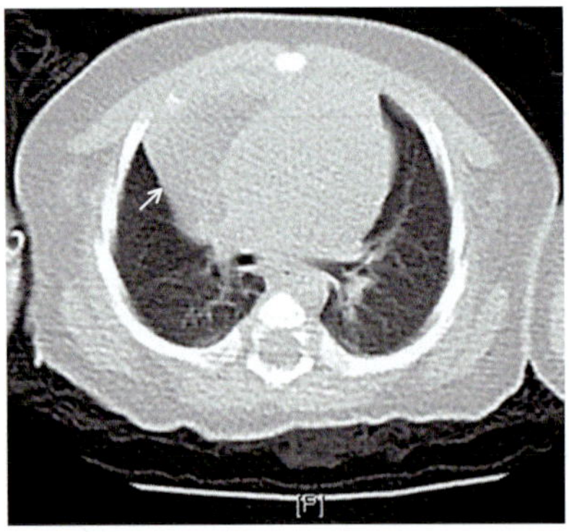

Fig. 10.9 A chest CT confirmed that the findings on the chest X-ray and lung ultrasound were caused by the thymus (*arrow*)

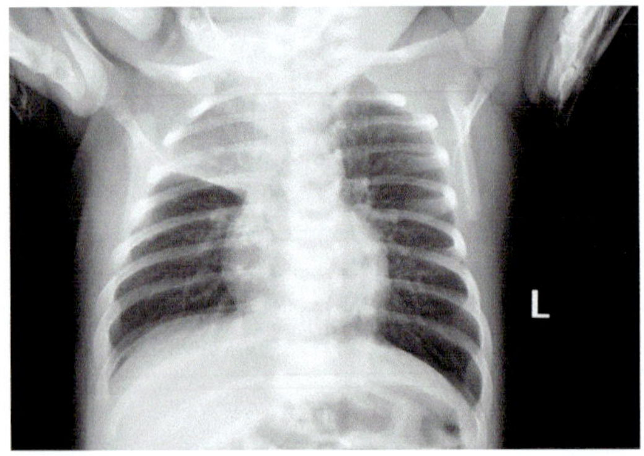

Fig. 10.10 A chest X-ray revealed atelectasis in the right upper lung

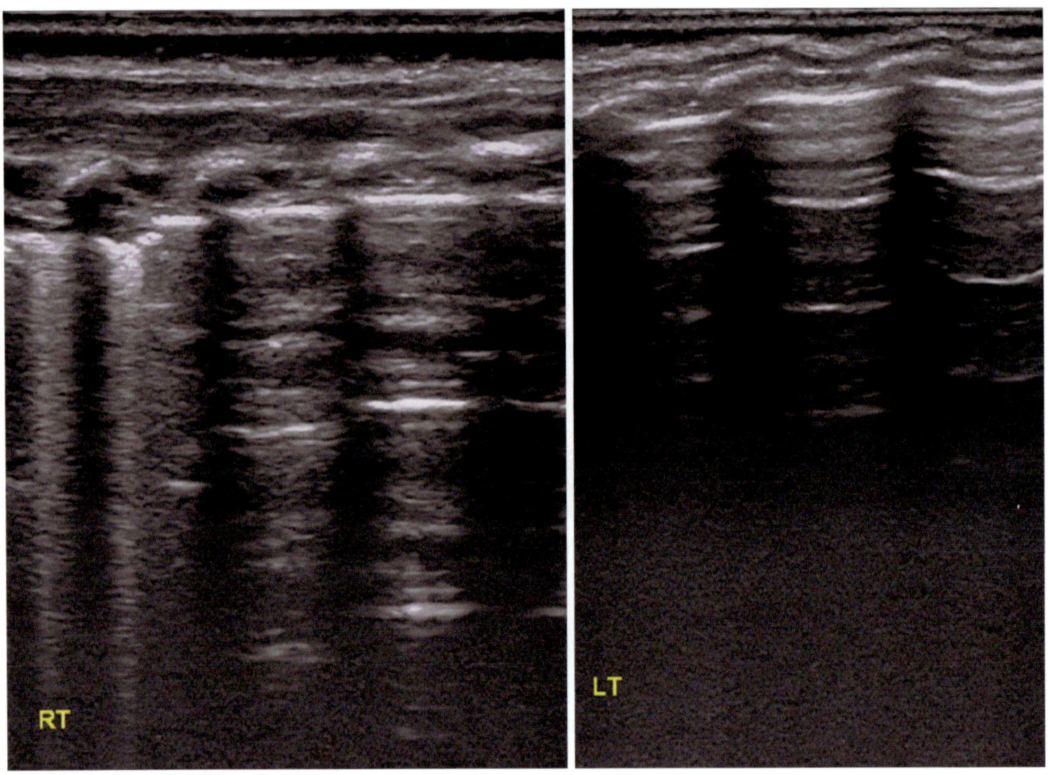

Fig. 10.11 A lung ultrasound (scanned from the patient's back) showed mild pneumonia in the right lung, while the left lung was normal

Case II: This was a male patient, G_1P_1, with a gestational age of 40 weeks, who was delivered vaginally and admitted to the hospital 22 days after birth because of mild pneumonia. A chest X-ray showed a large area of patchy, high-density shadows with clear edges in the right upper lung, which was suspected to be "right upper lung atelectasis" (Fig. 10.10). Lung ultrasound examinations performed by scanning the back of the baby showed subpleural focal lung consolidation in the right lung field with abnormal pleural lines, missing A-lines and AIS, while there were normal ultrasonographic findings in the left lung (Fig. 10.11). When the probe was

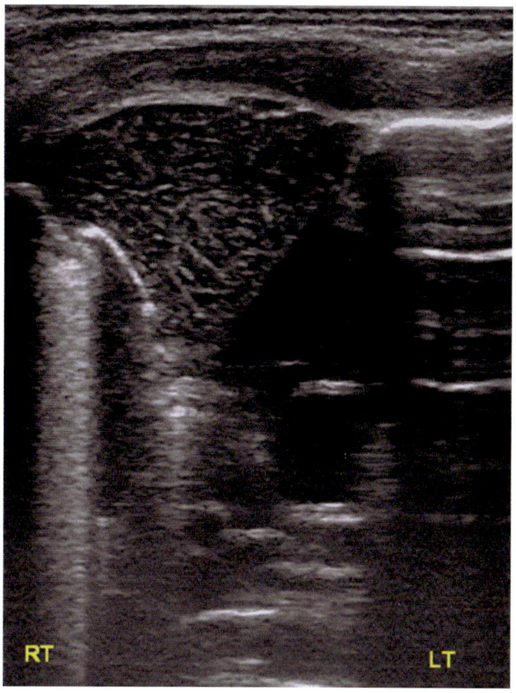

Fig. 10.12 A lung ultrasound (longitudinally scanned from the right front of midline) showed mild pneumonia in the right lung, while the left lung was normal

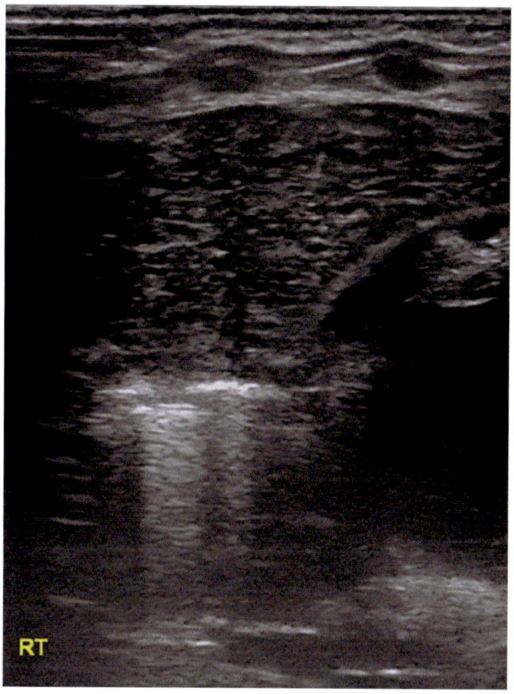

Fig. 10.13 An additional ultrasound examination from the anterior part of the chest confirmed that the large area of patchy, high-density shadow on the chest X-ray was the thymus

placed on the right lung and scanning was performed in a longitudinal direction, a dense medium echo shadow was visible in the right lung field above the heart, but there were normal pleural lines and A-lines in the left lung (Fig. 10.12). Further ultrasound examinations from the anterior part of chest confirmed that the large area of patchy, high-density shadow on the chest X-ray was mainly located in the middle mediastinum and right upper mediastinum (Fig. 10.13), and it was confirmed to be the thymus.

10.4 Lung Ultrasound More Accurately Reveals the Condition of Lung Diseases

Frequently, we found that chest X-rays revealed significant abnormal findings, but the lungs were actually normal clinically; thus, lung ultrasound might be useful in such conditions.

The patient was male, G_1P_1, with a gestational age of 40^{+3} weeks, who was delivered vaginally and had no asphyxia. He was admitted into the hospital 10 days after birth due to "difficulty breathing for 10 hours." On admission, the patient was diagnosed with "neonatal pneumonia" and placed on ventilator support based on his medical history, physical examination, lab tests, and chest X-ray. The patient was weaned off the ventilator 1 week later, and a chest X-ray revealed significant thickening and blurred lung markings with patchy, cloudy shadows. However, the patient was breathing steadily with clear breath sounds during lung auscultation and without any respiratory signs or symptoms. A lung ultrasound revealed clear, smooth, regular pleural lines and A-lines, and real-time ultrasound revealed pulmonary sliding. Some intercostal A-lines were unclear, and some B-lines were detected, with no consolidation, air bronchograms, or pleural effusion. Thus, the lung ultrasound was largely normal (Fig. 10.14) and was consistent with the clinical manifestations. Therefore, the patient was discharged.

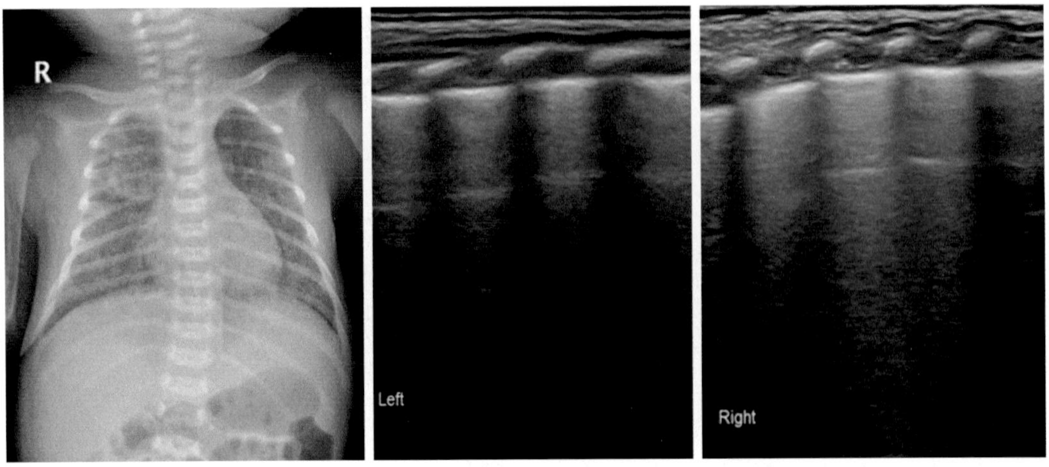

Fig. 10.14 A chest X-ray failed to accurately reveal the condition of the lungs. A chest X-ray revealed markedly increased and blurred lung markings, with significant patchy, cloudy shadows; however, a lung ultrasound revealed clear, smooth, regular pleural lines and A-lines. Thus, the ultrasound was normal, which was consistent with the clinical symptoms

10.5 Bronchoalveolar Lavage for the Treatment of Pulmonary Atelectasis, Severe Pneumonia, and MAS with Lung Ultrasound Monitoring

10.5.1 Pulmonary Atelectasis (PA)

Bronchoalveolar lavage (BL) has very good effectiveness for the treatment of neonatal pulmonary atelectasis when performed with lung ultrasound monitoring [3]. When a patient was diagnosed with PA via a pulmonary ultrasound examination, 1.5–3.0 mL of a saline or tracheal preservative solution (hereafter referred to as "lavage fluid") was intratracheally injected during each administration based on gestational age or body weight. If the pediatric patient was undergoing ventilator treatment, then the ventilator parameters were increased appropriately before the injection of the lavage fluid; specifically, the peak inspiratory pressure (PIP) was increased by 3–5 cmH_2O, the positive end-expiratory pressure (PEEP) was increased by 2–3 cmH_2O, the inspiratory time (Ti) was extended to 0.55–0.60 s, the respiratory rate (RR) was increased by 10–15 times/min, and the fraction of inspired oxygen (FiO_2) was increased appropriately based on the original ventilator parameters. After every injection of the lavage fluid, aeration was conducted for 10–20 mns, and then endotracheal intubation was performed under negative pressure to prevent sputum aspiration. Based on the degree of atelectasis, this suction was repeated 2–3 times per course of treatment. Depending on the disease condition of the pediatric patient, 1–2 courses of treatment were provided daily, and the requirement for reperfusion was determined later based on the lung recruitment status. For pediatric patients who did not receive ventilator treatment or were treated after weaning, intubation was needed again for endotracheal lavage, and positive pressure ventilation was performed using a resuscitation capsule or connection to a ventilator to assist the pediatric patients with breathing according to their individual conditions. After the end of each lavage course, a pulmonary ultrasound was immediately reviewed. The ultrasound findings were used to determine whether the next course of lavage and continuous ventilator treatment were needed [Figs. 10.15, 10.16, and 10.17].

10.5.2 Severe Pneumonia

In general, the major treatment for severe pneumonia is antibiotics and mechanical ventilation. We found that BL performed with lung ultra-

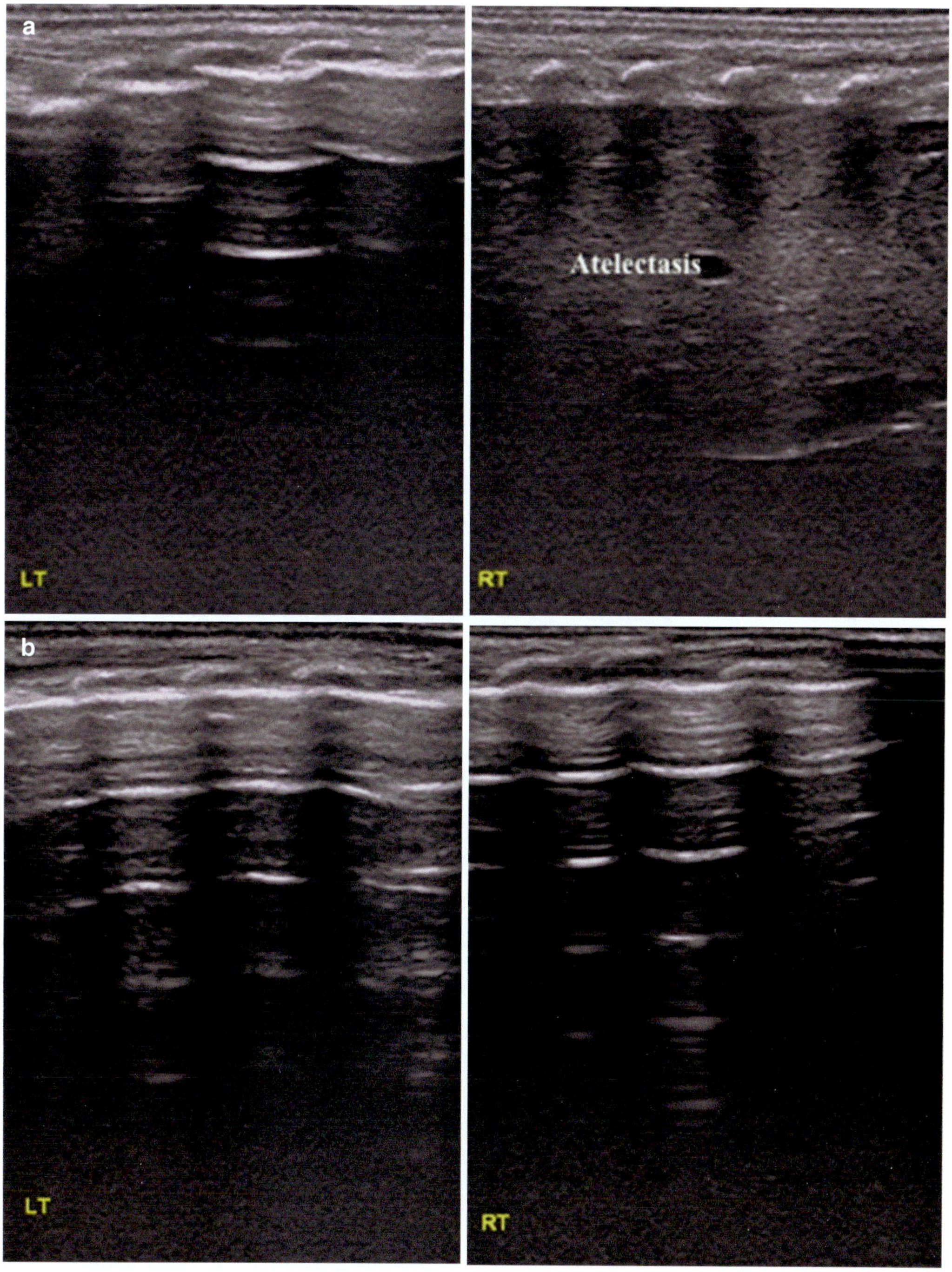

Fig. 10.15 (**a**) Before BL. (**b**) After BL. Severe PA affecting the entire right lung. A female patient with a gestational age of 37^{+4} weeks was admitted to the NICU due to severe asphyxia and MAS and was treated with ventilator support. Obvious dyspnea occurred after the ventilator was weaned 15 days later. A bedside LUS showed severe PA affecting the entire right lung (**a**). BL was provided immediately. After four cycles of lavage, recruitment was observed in the affected lung (**b**)

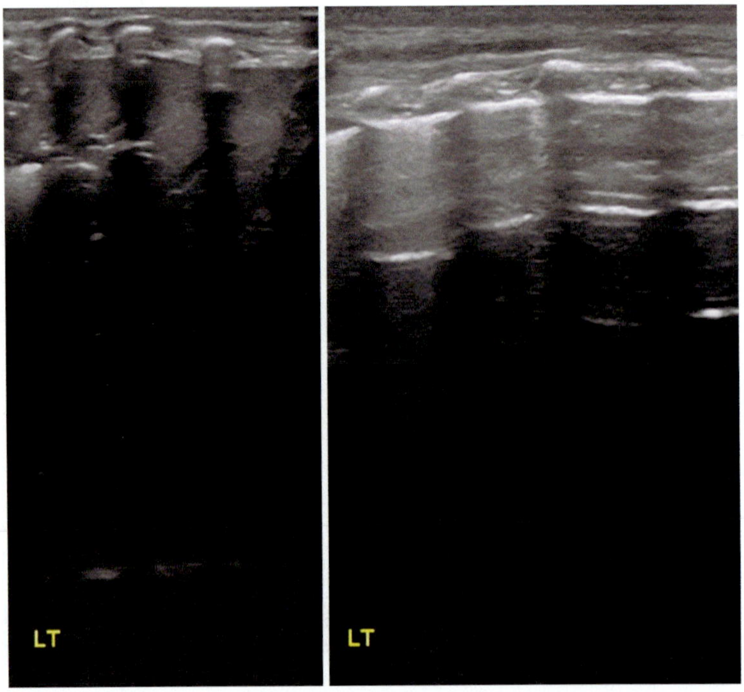

Fig. 10.16 Severe PA before (*left*) and after (*right*) BL. Severe PA in the left lung of a 38-week-old baby. The LUS showed severe PA (*left*). After one lavage treatment, recruitment was observed in the affected lung (*right*)

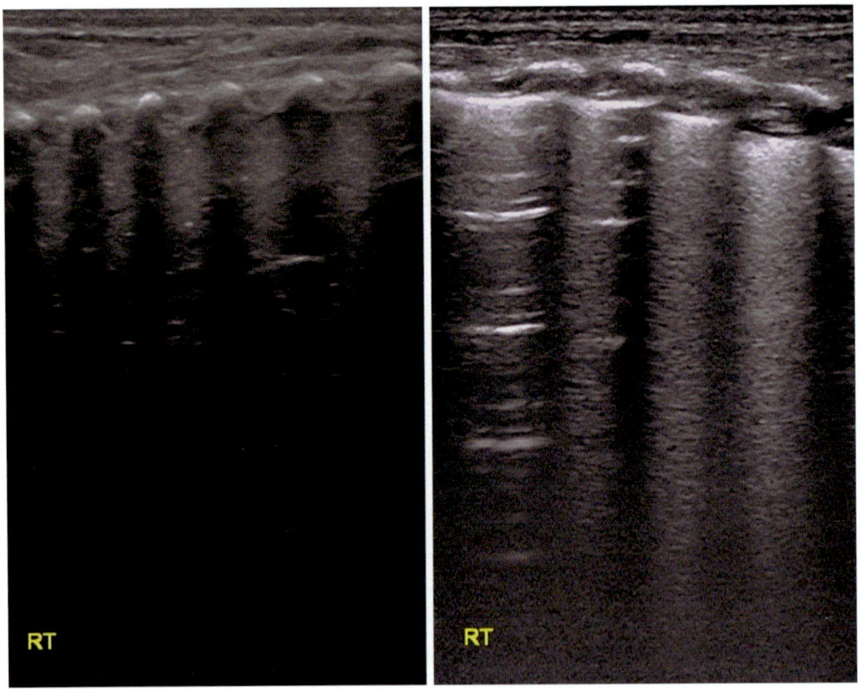

Fig. 10.17 Severe PA before (*left*) and after (*right*) BL. Severe PA in the entire right lung of a 38-week-old baby. A LUS showed severe PA affecting the entire right lung (*left*). After one lavage treatment, recruitment was observed, and only mild edema remained in the affected lung (*right*)

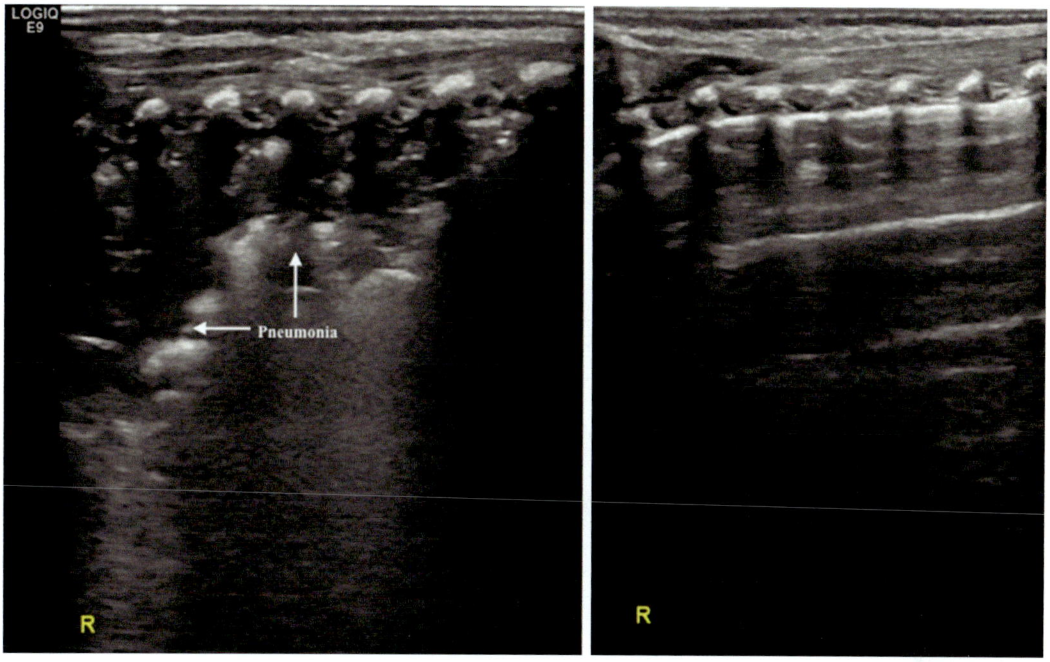

Fig. 10.18 Severe pneumonia (*left*) in the right lung of a 90-day-old baby with a gestational age of 27 weeks. During the treatment with antibiotics and ventilator support, BL was performed, and after several cycles of BL, the pneumonia completely resolved (*right*)

sound monitoring had good effectiveness for these patients, immediately decreasing the severity of the pneumonia and shortening the duration of mechanical ventilation and the length of hospital stay (Fig. 10.18).

10.5.3 BL for MAS

As previously described, MAS is one kind of lung disease of newborn infants, and severe MAS often requires treatment with mechanical ventilation for more than 10–14 days. We also found that BL performed with lung ultrasound monitoring has very good effectiveness for these patients and can significantly shorten the duration of mechanical ventilation and the length of hospital stay and even no need for continued ventilation in many patients.

This is a severe MAS patient with significant PA (Fig. 10.19a). The area of consolidation significantly diminished after two cycles of BL (Fig. 10.19b).

10.6 Thoracocentesis Drainage Performed with Lung Ultrasound Monitoring for Treating Neonatal PA Caused by Massive Congenital Pleural Effusion

PA caused by massive pleural effusion is rarely reported. Recently, a newborn infant with severe respiratory dyspnea was diagnosed with PA caused by massive congenital pleural effusion based on a lung ultrasound. Consolidated lung recruitment occurred after pleural puncture drainage with lung ultrasound monitoring.

This was a male baby with a gestational age of 38^{+6} weeks, a birth weight of 3870 g, no asphyxia at birth, and an Apgar score of 10, 10, and 10 at 1, 5, and 10 min after birth, respectively. This patient was hospitalized due to severe respiratory distress 3 h after birth. Physical examination revealed a full-term newborn appearance, significant thoracic distension, and respiratory distress manifested as a respira-

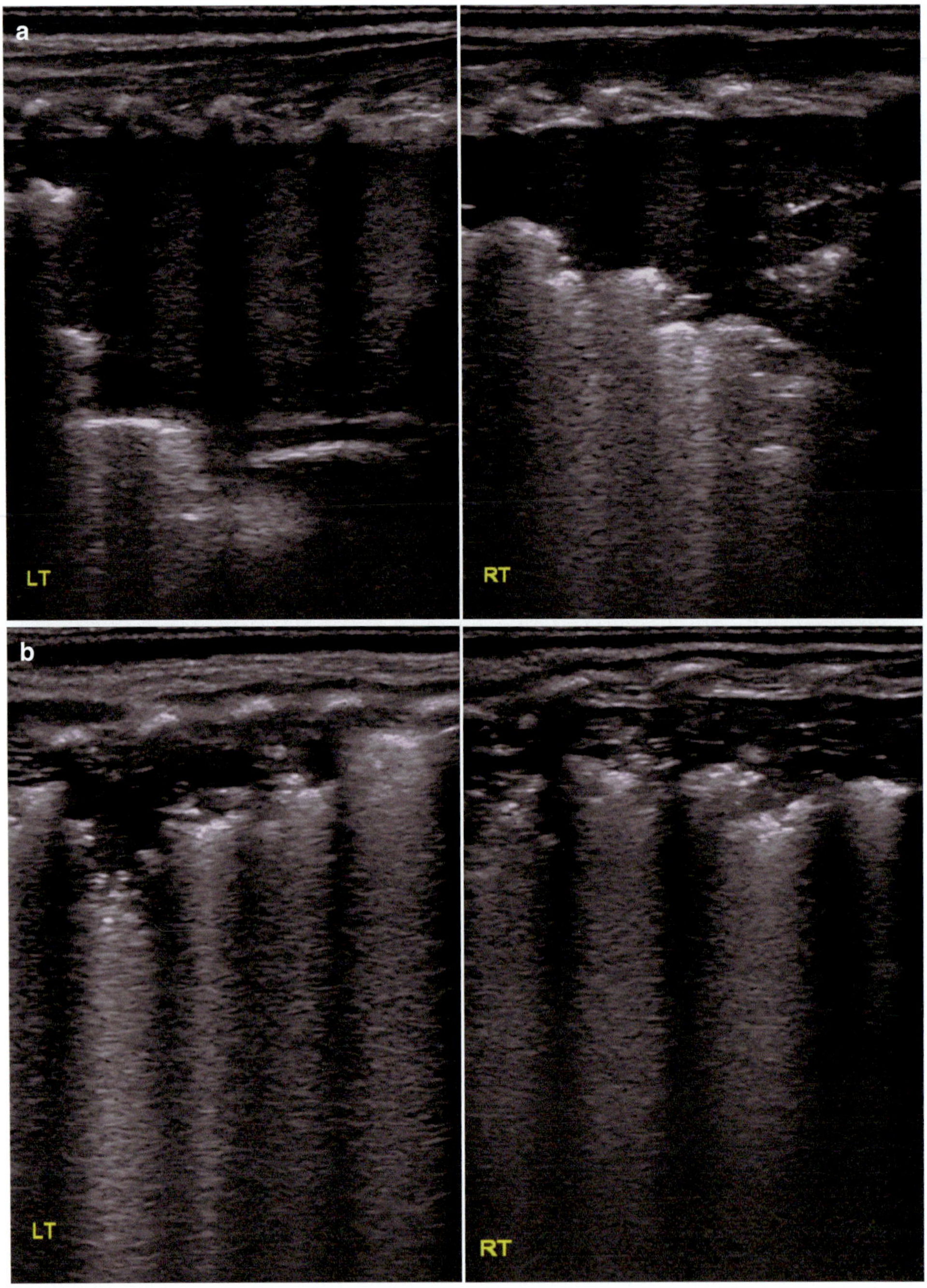

Fig. 10.19 (**a**) Before BL. (**b**) After BL

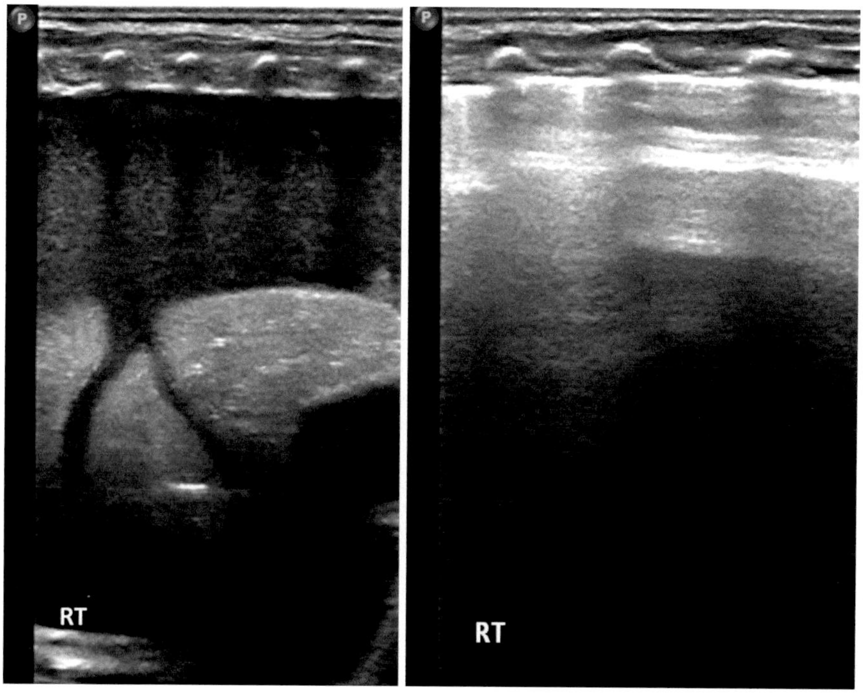

Fig. 10.20 Thoracic puncture for the treatment of atelectasis caused by massive pleural effusion. Thoracic puncture was performed in the right 5th-6th intercostal space along the posterior axillary line under ultrasound guidance. Lung recruitment of the consolidated and atelectatic lung occurred after 300 mL of flavescent fluid was drained. This picture shows the changes in the lung ultrasound before (*left*) and after (*right*) thoracic puncture

tory rate of more than 70 breaths/min accompanied by a restrictive respiratory pattern (Video 10.1). An ultrasound scan of the thorax showed a massive pleural effusion within the right hemithorax, and the three right lung lobes were compressed and contained dynamic air bronchograms that were visible with real-time ultrasound (Videos 10.2-1 and 10.2-2), which was confirmed to be atelectasis; however, the left lung was normal (Fig. 10.20, left). Thoracocentesis was performed at the right 5th-6th intercostal space along the posterior axillary line under ultrasonic guidance. Lung recruitment of the consolidated and atelectatic lung occurred after 300 mL of turbid fluid was drained (Fig. 10.20, right). The patient's difficulty breathing resolved after consolidated lung recruitment. The flavescent fluid was confirmed as a chylothorax with infection after routine and biochemical examinations.

10.7 Evaluating the Effectiveness of Exogenous Pulmonary Surfactant

1. Pulmonary surfactant (PS) often needs to be administered in severe lung disease, and ultrasonographic monitoring can accurately evaluate the efficacy of PS treatment. Generally, ultrasound monitoring should be performed within 2–3 h after PS is administered to the patient. After that, an ultrasound should be performed once every 12–24 h until ventilator withdrawal.
2. The prophylactic use of PS may be necessary for some extremely preterm infants, and an ultrasound should be performed before and within 1 h after PS is administered to the baby to observe any changes in the lung conditions; after that, monitoring should be performed once every 2–3 h after PS is administered to the baby until the possibility of RDS is ruled out.

References

1. Liu J, Chen SW, Liu F, et al. BPD, not BPD, or Iatrogenic BPD: findings of lung ultrasound examinations. Medicine. 2014;93(23):e133.
2. Liu J, Cao HY, Wang XL, et al. The significance and the necessity of routinely performing lung ultrasound in the neonatal intensive care units. J Matern Fetal Neonatal Med. 2016;29(24):4025–30.
3. Liu J, Ren XL, Fu W, et al. Bronchoalveolar lavage for the treatment of neonatal pulmonary atelectasis under lung ultrasound monitoring. J Matern Fetal Neonatal Med. 2017;30(19):2362–6.

MIX
Papier aus verantwortungsvollen Quellen
Paper from responsible sources
FSC® C105338

If you have any concerns about our products,
you can contact us on
ProductSafety@springernature.com

In case Publisher is established outside the EU,
the EU authorized representative is:
Springer Nature Customer Service Center GmbH
Europaplatz 3, 69115 Heidelberg, Germany

Printed by Libri Plureos GmbH
in Hamburg, Germany